SENSATIONAL KIDS SENSATIONAL FAMILIES

HOPE FOR SENSORY PROCESSING DIFFERENCES

PRAISE FOR SENSATIONAL KIDS, SENSATIONAL FAMÍLIES

"Just as the effects of wind can be seen without ever seeing the wind itself, so sensory processing disorder (SPD) presents in classrooms ... we can't see the disorder, but we see its effects through the seekers and avoiders who enter our room each year. Rebecca Duvall Scott's moving and honest memoir offers strategies not just for caregivers of children with SPD, but also for educators who desire to help support students with nervous system dysfunction like SPD and other pervasive developmental disorders. After trying many of the strategies in my kindergarten classroom, I saw behaviors begin to normalize and students become more ready to learn. This book shares information that could benefit veteran and new teachers alike."

Rebecca Wollam
Elementary School Teacher of the Year, 2018, Bullitt
County Public Schools, Louisville, Kentucky

"Through research and dedication Rebecca has performed what most people would consider to be impossible. I am so grateful that she is sharing her research and story with the world to bring hope and light to families in a time of frustration and darkness. As a healthcare provider and educator, I gained insight into the daily life of a family with a child who has sensory processing disorder, and I can't wait to start using what I have learned in my career and everyday life. Healthcare providers and educators are many times on the front-line caring for children who have nervous system dysfunction, and we can always deepen our awareness and sensitivity toward these children — as well as provide their families with answers and resources. I will be sharing this incredible story of hope to everyone who will listen!"

Jami Block, MSN-NE, APRN, NNP-BC

Advanced Practice Registered Nurse at Cincinnati Children's Hospital, certified Neonatal Nurse Practitioner, with a Masters of Science in Nursing Education and Currently Pursuing a PhD in the Healthcare Educators Program, Louisville, Kentucky

"Rebecca is insightful and determined in her unrelenting quest to parent her children; she has left no option unexplored. As a professional, traditional educator, I admire and respect her — and the beauty in her written words. Personally and professionally, we can all grow in our understanding that one size doesn't fit all kids — especially sensational kids."

Julie Cummings

Elementary Principal of the Year, 2017 and 2019, Jefferson County Public Schools, and Recipient of the Hilliard Lyons Principal Excellence Award, Louisville, Kentucky

"As Jacob's pediatrician, I witnessed personally this uplifting story of a mother's tenacity in her search for interventions to help her SENSATIONAL son. Rebecca leaves no stone unturned in her quest, including both mainstream and nontraditional therapies. WE can all learn from her willingness to try myriad remedies in pursuit of a happy, well-adjusted child. Her strategies may be of benefit to all parents of children with pervasive developmental disorders of all kinds."

Steve Kamber, MD, FAAP
Pediatrician, Partner of South Louisville Pediatrics, Louisville, Kentucky

"I started reading *Sensational Kids, Sensational Families* to learn more about Jacob's story ... only to discover through Rebecca's extensive research and personal experience that I was a sensory kid and am now a sensory adult. Thank you, Rebecca and Hannah, for giving meaning to something I've struggled with all my life! I not only recommend this book for parents with sensory kids; I recommend it for adults who are looking to understand why they're experiencing the world around them the way they do — and hopefully they'll find some possible antidotes."

Cathy Upshire
Wholeness Strategist, Author of *Woman Find Thyself* and *Evolution of a Woman*, Motivational Speaker and Wellness Coach, Founder of Broken Wings Coaching, LLC, — Helping Women Reclaim Their Sense of Identity and Power, Louisville, Kentucky

"We've worked through interventions with my special needs stepdaughter for more than 36 years with so many doctors. It was only through Rebecca's story, however, that I learned about sensory processing disorder. I wonder how many people suffer these challenges and never acquire the help they need. I marvel at all Rebecca and her family have done with Jacob, and I applaud her diligence and her generosity in writing this book!"

Annie Utick
Stepmother of a Special Needs Adult, Helena, Montana

"*Sensational Kids, Sensational Families* is a fascinating and inspiring book that taught me far more than I ever expected about the truly 'sensational' children and adults in my life. Rebecca's insights and stories – along with Hannah's professional deep-dives – helped me to better understand my own husband, who is a brilliant man with Asperger's syndrome (an autism spectrum disorder that includes among its hallmarks various sensory processing differences). After reading this book, I know two things for sure: 1) I am better equipped to support, understand and accommodate the sensational people in my personal and professional lives. 2) No matter what any of us are facing, there is a special kind of hope that reaps measurable results, and it starts with deep love, unflagging patience and the tenacity to keep fighting, even on the toughest of days. This book will change so very many lives for the better. What a gift!"

Kate Colbert
Aspie Wife, Dog Mommy, CEO and Author of *Think Like a Marketer: How a Shift in Mindset Can Change Everything for Your Business*, Kenosha, Wisconsin

"Rebecca and Hannah's book is prescriptive, not just for families affected by sensory processing disorder or pervasive development disorders, but for any parent who has had to swim upstream to advocate for their special needs child. Love-fueled persistence makes anything possible."

Lizbeth Meredith
Author of *Pieces of Me: Rescuing My Kidnapped Daughters*, Anchorage, Alaska

"From my experiences as a speech-language pathologist and a homeschooling mother, I can attest to how understanding sensory processing needs can help individuals reach their full potential. Rebecca's education, experience and passion are a great guide and encouragement to parents everywhere."

Rebecca Henderson
Former Speech Language Pathologist and Current Homeschooling Mom, Beaufort, South Carolina

"Rebecca Duvall Scott is an extraordinary mother who listened to her gut and refused to be dismissed when her concerns regarding behaviors and development were chalked up to 'he's a boy!' Her story is a sensational example of how the proper interventions and cohesive teamwork among medical providers, therapists and family can successfully improve the quality of life for someone living with sensory processing disorder."

Laurie Hellmann
Autism Mom and Author of *Welcome to My Life: A Personal Parenting Journey Through Autism*, Charlestown, Indiana

"As a former occupational therapist who worked in pediatrics and as a mother to both a teenage son with special needs and a neurotypical son, I can affirm that having a variety of sensory-based strategies and 'tools' is extremely beneficial. My oldest child has CHARGE Syndrome, a complex syndrome with extensive medical and physical challenges, which impacts how he processes and reacts to sensory information; therefore, we utilize several sensory based strategies with him daily. I even 'sneak in' some sensory activities for his neurotypical younger brother! *Sensational Kids, Sensational Families* offers real stories, struggles and — most importantly — more tools for my ever-evolving toolbox. It is also an amazing guide to utilize in teaching our kids how to meet their *own* sensory needs so they become functional, productive and happy adults. I highly recommend it to families and professionals alike."

Shawn Herrick
Former Occupational Therapist and Experienced Special Needs Mom, Louisville, Kentucky

"*Sensational Kids, Sensational Families* is a true gift! Rebecca, her son Jacob and their family's journey to find help will touch your heart in profound ways. As a mental health specialist and former educator, I've seen firsthand the vital need to break down existing stigmas surrounding behavior and diagnoses most often misunderstood. Rebecca will open your mind to better understand how we all uniquely process our world. This book, which leaves you equipped with compassion, knowledge, support and resources, offers hope for families, insight for professionals and will change the perspective of all who read it."

Penny Tate
Mental Health Specialist, Educator and Advocate, Antioch, Illinois

"Watching Jacob's story unfold — the trials, the victories and everything in between — helped give me confidence to try new ideas with my own son. I had never thought about how diet intervention could help modify behavior, but it has been life changing!"

Shannon McGrew
Mother of a Child with Attention Deficit Disorder
(ADD), Saint Mary's, Georgia

"What I love most about Rebecca's perspective is that rather than reacting to outward behavior, she encourages parents to be curious and discover the root of the underlying sensory issues. It's practical and personal, and will help many kids who today feel misunderstood."

Kirk Martin
Founder of CelebrateCalm.com, Fairfax, Virginia

"We all have the power to be sensational, and Rebecca's vulnerable memoir empowers everyone – whether personally touched by sensory processing disorder or not – to embrace what makes you *you* and learn ways to soar in life. As a parent of children who likely struggle with sensory differences, I was reminded by each word in this raw and welcoming book that there is beauty among the chaos and life among the confusion. With a dose of perspective paired with unwavering persistence, I now know that a diagnosis doesn't have to define you ... instead it can empower you!"

Stephanie Feger

Marketing Expert, Professional Speaker and Author of *Color Today Pretty: An Inspirational Guide to Living a Life in Perspective*, Louisville, Kentucky

"I applaud Rebecca for not giving up until she got to the bottom of Jacob's sensory issues. Some parents are so resistant to having their children tested or labeled. As a former teacher, I know it is a blessing to have a comprehensive and strategic plan to educate each child how they learn best and love them on their own terms."

Carla Griffin

Retired Elementary School Teacher at Goose Creek CISD, Highlands, Texas

"I found *Sensational Kids, Sensational Families* to be both honest and informative, written with an amazingly positive attitude that will act as encouragement to families facing similar sensational challenges. As a pediatric physical therapist, I love that Rebecca and Hannah were able to show the value of a strong parent/therapist team working together for the success of the child."

Jamie Ramsay

Pediatric Physical Therapist at Kids Center for Pediatric Therapies and Norton Children's Hospital, Louisville, Kentucky

"Rebecca Duvall Scott has provided the information and support I need. I realize I am not alone in parenting my son through sensory processing disorder; there are other people out there who completely understand!"

Amy Running

Private School Teacher, Tuscola County, Michigan

"I think Rebecca Duvall Scott's story is remarkable. I read how beautifully she writes each section and wonder if she realizes just how inspiring she is to so many. The love in her heart comes from above. Jacob was sent to Rebecca and Eric for a reason, and God is all around them. *Hope* is such an outstanding word, and this is what Rebecca is giving, not only to Jacob, but to the world!"

Brenda Miller

Vocalist in The Sherman Tomes Gospel Trio and Caretaker
of Siblings with Special Needs, Largo, Florida

"Rebecca Duvall Scott's personal testimony clearly shows that there aren't any quick fixes where sensory processing disorder is concerned, but it is a beautiful and challenging journey. It is honest, real, and hope-filled! What a great resource this book will be for many ... people can really trust Rebecca and Hannah with their loved ones!"

Pamela Leveritt

Independent Consultant at Arbonne International and Mother of an
Adult with Sensory Processing Disorder, La Grange, Kentucky

"I love Rebecca's outlook on life, parenting and this process with Jacob. It had to be super stressful at points, but she always circles back around to find the positive. Hooray for knowledge and great attitudes!"

Bonny Clapp

Mother of a Child with Autism, Murfreesboro, Tennessee

"On a personal level, I wish I'd had *Sensational Kids, Sensational Families* when my own son was going to occupational therapy every week for sensory processing challenges related to his obsessive-compulsive disorder. There is much here that could have helped me better understand my child and what he was experiencing. As an educator, this book is a reminder to meet students where they are, provide them choices (because not every child learns the same way, whether they have sensory processing disorder or not), be flexible, and see the entire child beyond whatever discipline you teach."

Carrie Vittitoe

Middle and High School Teacher at Educare Christian Cottage School and Jefferson County Public Schools, Creator of *Mood-Disordered Mama Blog*, and Podcast Host on *The Perks of Being a Book Lover*, Louisville, Kentucky

"Rebecca and her family have been on an inspiring journey. There is so much about child development that I knew nothing about until she sparked my interest. Her views on motherhood, parenting, and perseverance to improving one's experience are the embodiment of love. I hope she writes a sequel about the adolescent years!"

Mary Channon

Learning Management Systems Consultant, Chicago, Illinois

"I have seen firsthand the transformation that has come to Jacob and those who love him. We have been so fortunate to play a small role in his development. This wonderful exploration has only confirmed what I have known for years — that participating in Martial Arts can change lives. We look forward to implementing the knowledge contained in this book for the benefit of other students who struggle with sensory processing differences."

Master Mimi Hwang

Operations Director at Hwang's Martial Arts, Louisville, Kentucky

"I wish the whole world could read Rebecca's story. There are so many who need the encouragement only she can give."

Carol Duvall

Great-Aunt of a Child with Sensory Processing Disorder, Louisville, Kentucky

"I'm going to buy the additional books Rebecca has suggested — for myself and some of the close family — so I can get some support with this. I am grateful for her son's story and her ideas."

Emma Carpenter
Mother of Children with Autism and Sensory Processing Disorder, Ipswich, Suffolk, England

"As a parent, I believe it's through the resiliency of our children that we can learn the most. Rebecca and Jacob's journey is a testament to that belief. There is no doubt that their journey, so eloquently expressed on these pages, will impact the lives of many families who find themselves on similar, albeit unique paths in life."

Esther Ragan
Civil Servant and Community Advocate, Louisville, Kentucky

"A very timely, invaluable book for any parent raising a child with sensory processing disorder. The tools suggested by Rebecca Duvall Scott will empower families to restore health to their children, beginning with dietary changes that are foundational for healing the gut, immune and neurological systems. The blueprint outlined in this book has the amazing potential to allow many struggling children to lead normal, productive, healthy lives. A must read!"

Janet Pope, RN, BSN
Founding Member of Families for Effective Autism Treatment (FEAT) and Parent of an Amazing Young Man with Autism, Crestwood, Kentucky

SENSATIONAL KIDS
SENSATIONAL FAMILIES

HOPE FOR SENSORY
PROCESSING DIFFERENCES

REBECCA DUVALL SCOTT

WITH PROFESSIONAL COMMENTARY
BY OCCUPATIONAL THERAPIST
HANNAH RAGAN, MS, OTR/L

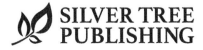

SILVER TREE
PUBLISHING

Sensational Kids, Sensational Families: Hope
for Sensory Processing Differences

By Rebecca Duvall Scott
With Professional Commentary by
Hannah Ragan, MS, OTR/L

Copyright 2020 by Rebecca Duvall Scott

Published by Silver Tree Publishing, a division of
Silver Tree Communications, LLC (Kenosha, WI),
under its Silver Linings Media imprint for memoirs.
www.SilverTreePublishing.com

Editing by:
Stephanie Feger
Kate Colbert

Cover design and typesetting by:
Lorenne Marketing & Design

First edition, March 2020

ISBN: 978-1-948238-27-4

Library of Congress Control Number: 2019920742

Created in the United States of America

Explanations, generalizations and advice in this book by Rebecca Duvall Scott with
professional commentary by occupational therapist, Hannah Ragan, are offered for
the sole purposes of sharing Jacob's personal journey and raising awareness about
sensory processing disorder (SPD). The authors are fully aware that SPD does not
have a diagnostic code in the Diagnostic and Statistical Manual of Mental Disorders
(DSM). Insights, recommendations, guidance and stories should not take the
place of professional and personalized medical advice or care for you, your loved
ones, your students, your clients or your patients. It is strongly recommended that
you consult with your own medical team regarding sequential steps in individual
diagnostic and treatment journeys, as each sensational person is unique in their
presentation of SPD and resulting needs.

DEDICATION

To my parents, family, numerous teachers and friends (all of whom believed in my writing when I was young, sitting in trees and making up stories); my husband and children who supported my dream of being a published author (even though the book was about them); and everyone who has joined "Team Jacob" and encouraged me to write this one-stop-shop kind of survival guide on sensory processing disorder... *Sensational Kids, Sensational Families*, my first and long-awaited published work, is for you — with so much love my heart could burst!

— *Rebecca Duvall Scott*

To all the individuals and families who struggle with sensory processing disorder daily, you are not alone. This book was written especially for you. May you find hope and new direction within these pages and the courage and grit needed to make your life sensational!

— *Hannah Ragan, MS, OTR/L*

CALLING *ALL* READERS: HOW TO KNOW IF THIS BOOK IS FOR YOU

FOR PARENTS, RELATIVES, SPOUSES, CARETAKERS OR FRIENDS OF A SENSATIONAL SOMEONE – THIS BOOK IS FOR YOU.

When sensory processing disorder (SPD) became a part of my family, I realized there was much to learn. To help others who find themselves connected to someone with SPD, this book explains the nuts and bolts of the disorder and is jam-packed with intervention strategies that can improve your loved one's functioning and quality of life, no matter what age. My candid story shouts from the rooftop that **YOU ARE NOT ALONE**! As you read on, you will discover what many wish they had known all along, including myself when I was in your shoes.

FOR THERAPISTS, TEACHERS, PSYCHOLOGISTS OR PROFESSIONALS WITH SENSATIONAL CLIENTS AND STUDENTS – THIS BOOK IS FOR YOU.

My goal is to empower you with a better understanding of the elusive world of SPD through my tell-it-like-it-is description of life with a sensational person. Whether you engage with individuals diagnosed with SPD in a home setting, office or classroom, you can take the knowledge and strategies I've utilized and adapt them to fit your work, an effort which will be rewarded tenfold. **BE BRAVE** enough to break the mold and start changing lives, one sensational child at a time.

FOR DOCTORS, NURSES OR MEDICAL PROFESSIONALS WITH SENSATIONAL PATIENTS – THIS BOOK IS FOR YOU.

The understanding of sensory processing and how it manifests and affects all aspects of life elevates this book above the knowledge of medical practices that are still controlled by reaction, rather than prevention. I know this because I've lived this. For the health of your clients through quicker diagnoses and referrals to therapy, please take the time to read on. Let my family's medical discoveries be a catalyst in your career to dig deeper, learn more and treat sensational people with the **BEST METHODS** available.

IF YOU, YOURSELF, ARE SENSATIONAL – THIS BOOK IS FOR YOU.

You may have lived your whole life feeling different, more or less, than your peers. If you see yourself in these pages, let hope float. Sensory processing and nervous system functioning can be improved, one day at a time, in many different ways — no matter your age! Learn how to minimize your weaknesses and maximize your strengths, and **BE PROUD** of who you are. Not all of us are truly sensational.

IF YOU ARE A NAYSAYER AND BELIEVE ALL MISBEHAVIOR IS A DISCIPLINE ISSUE — YES, THIS BOOK IS FOR YOU, TOO!

You may have people in your personal circle that you think are odd, or children you're *sure* just need proper discipline. Discipline is vital, but I know firsthand that it doesn't fix everything. I implore you to read this book and be open to a new perspective, supported by both research and science. The people you think are "weird" and kids you think are just "troublemakers" may actually be **SENSATIONAL** if you give them a chance.

WRITE YOUR OWN STORY

When they said something was wrong with you, I grieved.
I questioned, "Can this be fixed? Will he grow out of it?"
Hope broke like delicate crystal;
It slipped out of my grip and shattered in all directions.
Then, just as quickly, came Faith and Determination.
I picked up the shards, the sharp edges cutting my hands —
This would not be our story.

I fought for you.
I still fight. Every day, we rise.
Battling against disbelief, ignorance, the unknown ...
Striving to heal your body and mind, to mirror that
God-given soul, beautiful in its perfection.
With God, we will write our own words.

I look at your sweet face, that knowing grin, those bright eyes.
I cherish the blessings this journey holds.
Battles fought, lost and won, leave in the wake
A better family, a fiercer love, an embrace of what matters.
Hope reflects off every piece that was broken.
Hope lights up the room.
This will be our story ... the one we write together.

— Rebecca Duvall Scott

TABLE OF CONTENTS

PART THREE
Attitudes That Made the Difference 117

PART FOUR
The After-Story and Acknowledgments........... 175

PART FIVE
Resources to Aid You on Your Journey 201

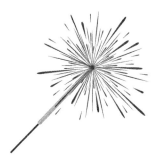

PART ONE

THE BACKSTORY

THE SCOTT FAMILY

Eric and I were college sweethearts. We married two weeks after graduation, both of us very proud to graduate among the top of our class and to be the first college graduates in our respective families. We set off to build our lives with enduring love and hard work. He was all things math, and I was all things English ... two halves of the whole.

I've been writing since I was small, and being a published author was always the end-goal. It was my dream. I won writing contests at local, county and state levels through my K-12 years, and I went on to write the first 70 pages of a novel for a creative writing class in college. But as it does to each of us, life happened. I laid my writing on a shelf in favor of being a behavioral interventionist for children with autism, then left that important work to be a wife, and finally my most rewarding job — a mother. I always imagined my first book, when I got back around to writing, would be the novel I had started in college. Publishing a "self-help" style memoir about special needs never entered my mind.

Eric and I were just enjoying the life we built together. He went to work and brought home the bacon, and I kept the house and children. Most people think us old-fashioned, but, to us, we are just a good old love story at its finest.

Eric and I were just enjoying the life we built together. He went to work and brought home the bacon, and I kept the house and children. Most people think us old-fashioned, but, to us, we are just a good old love story at its finest.

It's important for you to know us, because *we* start the story. Before there was sensory processing disorder (SPD), there was just sweet Jacob. Before Jacob, darling Annabelle. And before Annabelle, Eric and Rebecca — newlyweds with so much living to do.

Our first born, Annabelle, is a deeply sensitive, emotional and intelligent "old-soul." I had worked with so many autistic clients who used American Sign Language (ASL) to communicate that I learned the basic signs for babies and was gung-ho to try it out on my own daughter. She was signing back well before her first birthday, and rarely had tantrums or meltdowns — even in the stereotypical terrible twos. By then, she was verbal and talking buckets of words. She could also work a 25-piece United States puzzle by herself... at age 2 1/2 . I hid outside the playroom and watched her do it, making sure there wasn't a puzzle-working ghost in the house! She continues to excel in everything she puts her mind to, scoring well above her grade level on standardized tests and impressing us as she rises to the occasion at every turn. She is my predictable and safe-choice kid, my reliable rock of a helper in so many ways. It's important for you to know her, too, for she is an integral part of our story ... my persistent and perfectionist daughter who adds a rainbow to any downcast day.

Next comes Jacob, our second-born. As I was writing this book he frequently would ask, "Am I the star?" Most of the time I would say, "No," explaining that the book is about sensory processing disorder and the hard work we did — him, me, Dad, Sister, all of us. But sometimes I'd look into those twinkling eyes and say, "Yes, you *are* the star." We've raised both our children to know their worth, that they are both special beyond words, but we've also raised *him* to know he is sensational. It matters a great deal to Jacob, especially, that our story be told.

It matters a great deal to Jacob, especially, that our story be told.

Even after all the interventions and progress, Jacob is still our impulsive, thrill-seeking and wonderfully hilarious boy. He is our energetic, vivacious, live-in-the-moment kid. It took us a *long* time to get here. He was an easy-going baby until around a year old. Even then, I thought the change was *me* and not him. You see, that was when I had spinal fusion surgery to repair a pinched nerve from my pregnancy, which physical therapy couldn't fix. After my surgery, I needed extra help around the clock. Annabelle was 3 and Jacob was just turning 1. I could not lift them, bathe them, stand and fix their lunches, rock them to sleep — nothing. For quality time during my recovery, they laid in bed next to me as I held a book up and read to them. I worked hard to rehabilitate my body, but two months without being the primary caregiver took its toll on the kids. Jacob especially had grown to be distressed in many ways, and I blamed the spikes in his energy and aggression on the major routine changes that took place after my surgery. It never got back to normal, however, no matter what I did.

My mom, who is like my right-hand man, kept saying, "What is going on with Jacob? He's getting worse. His behavior is getting a lot worse." She was one of his two Sunday School teachers, and because he could level the room faster than they could catch him, she affectionately nicknamed him "Captain Destructo" ... as only a Mamaw can get away with.

My mom, who is like my right-hand man, kept saying, "What is going on with Jacob? He's getting worse. His behavior is getting a lot worse." She was one of his two Sunday School teachers, and because he could level the room faster than they could catch him, she affectionately nicknamed him "Captain Destructo" … as only a Mamaw can get away with.

Jacob lived up to his nickname, though. For two years, Eric and I tag-teamed him and each took shifts on "Jacob Duty." One parent cared for him solely as he would literally hang from the curtains, climb the walls, and dump and destroy anything and everything in sight. The other parent rested and took care of calm, quiet, sweet Annabelle. I knew in my heart something was going wrong, but I couldn't put my finger on what it was. I ruled out autism. I had worked with many children with that developmental disorder and knew he didn't have enough indicators, so *what* was making him unmanageable?

I was becoming increasingly unsettled; the panic only a suspecting mother knows rising with the tide. He was 3 years old at the time, and doctor after doctor answered my behavioral concerns with: "He's just 100% boy and within normal developmental range. Don't compare him to his sister." The scary part of the story is that if it wasn't for me pushing the pediatrician for a speech therapy evaluation (he babbled continually but was rarely understood — which added to the chaos and confusion), we would have lost precious, critical years of our story.

Thankfully, once I connected him with a speech pathologist, the right path organically unfolded for Jacob. When the speech therapist offered an explanation, I jumped at the opportunity for knowledge. She suspected SPD, and it was her recommendation to get him evaluated by occupational therapy, another branch of therapy that could potentially help him *calm down*. I didn't know why or how, but "calm" sure sounded good to this momma's harried soul. She gave me a photocopied pamphlet, which offered some basic information about SPD, within the subtype of "sensory-seekers." I read it at the stop lights on the way home. The description might as well have had Jacob's picture next to it! I felt an odd sensation of having gripped a life-preserver, yet I was still too far out in the ocean for it to make a difference. I like to have a plan, after all. I like to know where to go from here … and I hadn't a clue how to pull myself to shore. What exactly was SPD? What would it mean for Jacob and our family? Would he grow out of it or learn to live with it? Will he always be this way? What caused it in the first place? Was there a root cause?

I felt an odd sensation of having gripped a life-preserver, yet I was still too far out in the ocean for it to make a difference.

Eric, who was supportive of my efforts to explore SPD and occupational therapy, still pressed quietly, "I just want to understand *why* he is more than 100% boy. What is he doing that is actually atypical?" Well, for starters Jacob was wild as a little buck. We really were just doing our best to corral this bundle of intense, vibrating energy that could jet around the house, store, church or park at Mach speed, leaving a wake of destruction in his path. Once, at a family birthday party, he went careening through our house from the bedroom to the kitchen (squealing all the way like an incoming jet plane), bumping into walls and people's legs, pulling one cousin's hair as he flew past, and grabbing the baby cousin around the neck and carrying her several feet like a dangling, choking teddy bear with bulging eyes. I had read James Dobson's *Bringing Up Boys*, which likened boys to cars, having all gas and no steering. If that was typical 100% boys, Jake was about 500%! He not only was all gas and no steering, but he also had a flat tire, smoking engine, and exhaust pipe dragging the ground that left a spray of sparks! Lack of impulse control was a gross understatement. He was a force that could *not* be reckoned with. He was a mini-tornado, with beautiful eyes and a sweet wind-me-up-and-watch-me-go smile!

You know what most people think? I'm making excuses for a child who just needed more *discipline*. I am well acquainted with the criticism and advice from people who have never lived with, or tried to raise, an SPD kiddo, and I have grown thick skin because of it. Even though he was not typically rude, mean or hateful (thank goodness), we openly admit he was a handful. In the grocery store, we were the family on the receiving end of glares and negative whispers. Jacob would be in the cart, riding along, and when we steered too close to the shelves, he would reach and rake boxes and cans off — clapping and squealing with joy at the clattering mess. We would start keeping tabs on his hands, but somehow when we took our eyes off of him for a second, his toes could reach where his fingers could not and there would be more havoc.

I am well acquainted with the criticism and advice from people who have never lived with, or tried to raise, an SPD kiddo, and I have grown thick skin because of it.

His mouth was also never quiet. When he tired of sitting, he would continue babbling and squealing as he would escape from the seatbelt and slither out of the cart like an octopus. We would try to pry him from the cart mid-attempt to reseat him, but every time we got his hands free, his toes held on, and when we got his toes free, his hands would find another stronghold. Then the wailing would begin. There is no consoling a tired and irritable child who has been in the store past their limit. We would continue to desperately stuff his tentacles back in the cart, simultaneously getting our top priority shopping done, and we'd attempt to get out of there with a little of our energy and dignity intact. Even with my behavioral therapy background and knowing in my heart this was not a result of faulty parenting, I still wondered why I could not rein him in.

And in case you're wondering, we *did* spank him from time to time, and we did more than our fair share of time-outs and loss of privileges ... I am telling you: NOTHING WORKED.

And in case you're wondering, we *did* spank him from time to time, and we did more than our fair share of time-outs and loss of privileges ... I am telling you: NOTHING WORKED.

Nothing dialed the energy level down, or even gave him the slightest pause before he'd engage in another misbehavior. If anything, physical discipline actually made things *worse*. I was exhausted trying to figure out how to help him "be good." That's another reason I'm so thankful someone told me about SPD before long-term damage was done to his self-esteem. It's like one moment I was stumbling in the dark, and then the light flipped on. SPD was a family-saving diagnosis. It gave us new direction, an action plan to help him, and — most importantly — it helped us teach Jacob how to help himself!

SPD was a family-saving diagnosis.

When our story began, I had no idea that our journey to heal and appreciate Jacob's SPD challenges would end up touching so many lives. It changed us for the better — individually and collectively. If you or someone you love are fighting a similar battle, I truly hope that within the coming pages you can begin to see the forest for the trees as I did and gather the strength and courage it takes to bring a brighter future within reach. Sensory challenges, from slight to severe, can be managed. We did it. You can, too.

Sensory challenges, from slight to severe, can be managed. We did it. You can, too.

Mrs. Hannah Ragan

I am Hannah Ragan, and I was Jacob's occupational therapist for almost four years. I received my Master's in Occupational Therapy in 2009 and have found it fulfilling to help the many individuals who come through my office. My experience in pediatric occupational therapy comprises work with the public school systems, outpatient transitional rehab, and early intervention home health services. In these settings, I have performed evaluation and treatment of neurological and orthopedic patients with a variety of diagnoses, including but not limited to: cerebral palsy, spina bifida, brachial plexus injuries, central nervous system dysfunction, sensory and regulatory disorders, attention deficit hyperactivity disorder, learning disorder, pervasive developmental disorders, developmental delay, oppositional defiant disorder, autism, Asperger's syndrome, Norrie disease, Sotos syndrome, Down syndrome, cerebrovascular accident, brain injury, and Prader-Willi syndrome.

My certifications include Interactive Metronome, Beckman Oral Motor Assessment and Intervention, and Physical Agent Modalities, including Neuromuscular Electrical Stimulation and Reiki I. Furthermore, I am certified to implement craniosacral therapy with both adults and children, and I have acquired Level I training in Neurokinetic Therapy. I also regularly complete continuing education training on sensory integration/processing, and I educate occupational therapy students from accredited occupational therapy programs in the field.

Over the years, Rebecca and Jacob have impressed upon me their passion and drive, evoking a high level of respect for their commitment to meeting both SPD, and life, head on.

Over the years, Rebecca and Jacob have impressed upon me their passion and drive, evoking a high level of respect for their commitment to meeting both SPD, and life, head on.

I remember first meeting Rebecca and her son, Jacob, then just 3 years old. I see many children with sensory processing disorder (SPD), along with their parent(s)/guardian(s), but Rebecca left a distinct impression on me. Her preparation for our initial session was extensive and thorough. She presented me with a meticulous journal, which recorded Jacob's behaviors in response to stimuli, in conjunction with the length of time it took to calm certain behaviors utilizing various sensory strategies, such as pushing/pulling or other movement activities. As a therapist who works predominantly with children presenting with special needs, I recognize the importance of working equally as close with their caregivers. Progress gained in therapy is often as much dependent on the primary caregiver as it is on the skill of the therapist. Thus, a caregiver such as Rebecca — who is well informed, devoted and an active participant on the home front — is both a precious gift to the child and the participating therapist.

Jacob, or "the little bulldozer" as I dubbed him (due to his enthusiasm and boundless energy from our initial session), is as bright as he is energetic. My favorite memory of our time together was when Jacob and I were focusing on the consequences of one's actions. With any child, but particularly with Jacob, this was a challenging and continuous lesson. On one occasion, he left the therapy gym in very low spirits, because he had hit me and, as a result of his actions, he didn't get to play in the coveted ball pit. Soon after, Jacob's sister accompanied him to a therapy session, and I asked Jacob to explain our facility's gym rules to her, assuming Jacob would recite the general rules. I was surprised when I heard Jacob solemnly inform his sister of one rule: "We don't hit Miss Hannah." In that moment, Jacob solidified his place in my heart. He had taken the lesson we had worked so diligently on and applied it in a very serious and intense way.

Throughout this book, Rebecca paints a vivid and authentic picture of what it is like raising a child with SPD. You will be drawn into the joys and hardships of their journey from the moment of Jacob's diagnosis, to the experiences surrounding the exploration of Jacob's treatment options, and their hard-earned success. As a therapist, I believe this story is beneficial not only to fellow parents, but teachers and health-care professionals as well. Rebecca is a caregiver who not only applies methods of treatment she is presented with but expounds upon them to achieve maximum results.

I find Rebecca's research and experiences to be an ideal guide for those who are just beginning their journey and for those already traveling on the path searching for hope. For additional understanding and support, I also share my professional opinion throughout the book on commonly asked questions regarding SPD. I highly recommend this book as a tool to combat SPD from all angles.

UNDERSTAND SPD AND GET EARLY INTERVENTION

Let's dig in: What *is* sensory processing disorder (SPD)? To understand the disorder, you first have to understand sensory processing and what it does for every person. A well-functioning nervous system is responsible for processing incoming information from the senses (mainly using the five basic senses of sight, hearing, smell, taste and touch — and two less-known senses of vestibular/movement and proprioceptive/pressure, among others). Your brain receives sensory information from your environment, decides what is important or what to disregard, and then sends out behavioral responses to keep you functioning appropriately within your environment. If music is too loud and hurts your ears, you turn it down. If walking in the grass drives you crazy, you put on shoes. You spin on a merry-go-round until you've had enough, and you get off before you hurl. The party is getting wild and you either excuse yourself to go home and watch a movie in your sweatshirt, or you jump at the chance to become the life of it. Input sensory information — output behavioral response. We each do it every day, all day long. We just don't *realize* it.

Input sensory information — output behavioral response. We each do it every day, all day long. We just don't *realize* it.

Every person has sensory preferences, things they like and don't like, but where it becomes a disorder is when the preferences or needs keep you from functioning properly. A true sensory disorder means that your nervous system is malfunctioning. For some reason or another, it does not process sensory input correctly. Lights become too bright. Regular noise levels become unbearably loud. Clothes become scratchy and cumbersome. Regular food becomes horribly unappealing to the point of gagging and vomiting. Modulation of force, energy and more spins hopelessly out of control. It *inhibits* you living life.

Sensory processing, or sensory integration, was first defined by occupational therapist, Jean Ayres in 1972 as "the neurological process that organizes sensation from one's own body and from the environment and makes it possible to use the body effectively within the environment."[1] Therefore, if your sensory system is malfunctioning, your brain is misinterpreting the information coming into your body, or cannot organize it properly, thus it cannot output appropriate responses.

SPD manifests in a variety of ways, but there are two main categories, like two sides of the same coin: avoiders and seekers. A person with SPD is dominantly one or the other, but the lines can get blurred from day to day. It is normal for people with SPD to show traits of both categories, which makes the disorder that much more confusing and slippery to get a grip on.

---

1   Marie E. DiMatties, "Understanding Sensory Integration," http://www.ldonline.org/artlcle/5612/

SPD manifests in a variety of ways, but there are two main categories, like two sides of the same coin: avoiders and seekers.

Avoiders are the ones who readjust their socks a million times (or just buy seamless socks), cut tags out of clothing or only wear a limited wardrobe, have a very self-restricted diet of foods, cover their ears in loud places, refuse to go into public bathrooms for fear of toilets flushing, need sunglasses in the house, and typically feel an intense need to control their environment so they feel prepared and safe. If their expectations are violated, they can go 0-60 mph in less than a minute! Every sensation is too much to handle, because they are so sensitive to stimuli. Therefore, we say avoiders have *hypersensitive* sensory systems.

In contrast, **seekers** have *hyposensitive* sensory systems ... they seem to crave input but can never get enough. These are the kids who don't stop moving from dawn until dusk, and then wiggle or rock themselves to sleep. They don't sleep much and, during the waking hours, they are a force to be reckoned with. They bump, crash, jump, slam, scream, twirl, bang, hit, kick ... these are the kids who get labeled as behavior cases, because they seemingly cannot be controlled. If they have SPD, however, the reason for their behaviors is that their "sensory bucket" doesn't get filled up properly from everyday activities that satiate the rest of us. Therefore, they seek input any way they can, often in raucous and socially inappropriate ways.

Both categories of sensory system dysfunction — avoiders and seekers — carry stigma. Too often, avoiders are called sissies or melodramatic, and seekers are considered obstinate and defiant. Both scenarios are often assumed to be due to faulty parenting, adding insult to injury. The truth, however, is that SPD is a hidden medical condition — like fibromyalgia. People may not be able to see it on the outside, but these kids' nervous systems are malfunctioning. They cannot generally help their behavior without intervention, much like sick people need medicine to feel well.

The good news is that SPD can be managed, and sometimes even healed to the point the diagnosis is no longer valid.

The good news is that SPD can be managed, and sometimes even healed to the point the diagnosis is no longer valid.

While I was waiting for an evaluation with an occupational therapist (OT), I kept researching. I had filled out the paperwork the therapy center had mailed me, and because I didn't feel like the checklist of symptoms even scratched the surface of what we were dealing with, I also wrote a lengthy observation on the back of the forms about life with Jacob at home. I needed to share details with them such as how he wiggled himself to sleep at night, slept for a few precious hours that were fraught with intermittent waking, and woke up like a rocket. I was very nervous about how the evaluation would go, and most of all how *bad* they would say he was. I wanted answers but, then again, I was worried the truth would change our lives in ways I wasn't prepared for.

Eric and I sat in a little office while the OT doing the evaluation asked us a bazillion questions and Jacob roamed the room. He rummaged through a few shelves of toys that were within reach, and then tried to climb the bookshelf. She redirected him to the table and tried to engage him in various peg-hole puzzles and toys that screwed together. He pushed them away, stood up on the bench and jumped off onto a mat in the corner. He entertained himself while looking at his reflection in a mirror, and every time he heard the workmen outside the window, he would get flustered and repeatedly ask, "What's that?" until he understood that the new sounds were nothing to fear. We talked, with the therapist observing Jacob's behavior and interaction for the better part of the hour, and then she tried to get him to sit again and use a pencil to copy a few simple lines and shapes. He pushed the pencil to the paper as hard as he could, his little fist turning white as he strangled it. He managed to scratch a few quick marks before abruptly lifting it with an upswing that nailed the therapist square in the nose! I wanted to crawl under my chair.

We apologized for his unruly behavior, especially when he blew a raspberry in her face and jumped off the bench to play in front of the mirror again. I felt sick to my stomach. I wanted to scoop him up and leave. It seemed easier to just go back to struggling, day by day, on my own than to wonder what this professional thought of him and us. New people and places absolutely brought out the worst in Jacob, but this evaluation took the cake! I honestly didn't know how the OT would draw any conclusions from such a noisy, anxious, disjointed visit. She had seen all she needed to draw plenty of conclusions, though ... and they were surprisingly spot-on.

Jacob's official assessment, using "The Sensory Processing Measure - Preschool (SPM-P)," scored him in the *Some Problems* range for social participation, balance and motion scales, and in the *Definite Dysfunction* range on the vision, hearing, touch, body awareness, planning and ideas scales. Ouch. I read that report several times, but I didn't understand most of it. I had no idea what it meant for him or for us as a family. I just understood the *some problems* that led to the painful *definite dysfunction*. It was a punch in the gut to have someone of trusted authority confirm that there was something "wrong" with our child, but the worst part was that I didn't know how we were going to "fix" him. I, for one, felt powerless. That's when my own proactive behavioral therapist attitudes came back to me.

Many times, I had said to autism clients with new diagnoses: "Don't get stuck in denial, but dig in and work hard for change, one day at a time." Now it was my turn to be brave.

Many times, I had said to autism clients with new diagnoses: "Don't get stuck in denial, but dig in and work hard for change, one day at a time." Now it was my turn to be brave.

In most cases, early intervention is a vital key in treating nervous system disorders. The nervous system is very malleable (or moldable) in the formative years, so the more changes you can make early-on the better; it gets more difficult to change nervous system functioning as a person ages. I *knew* that. So, Eric and I put grief and uncertainty behind us as quickly as possible and turned our attention to building a successful future. It was time to research, make a plan, execute it one day at a time, and start moving forward again. The stalemate between us and SPD had lasted long enough; I was going after my boy.

I worked with a scheduler at the therapy center to get us started in weekly OT. We talked on the phone several times, trying to find a person who could fit us in, and when it came down to the fourth phone call to discuss two possible therapists, I finally told her, "I don't know these people like you do. Our life is in your hands. All I can tell you is how I need someone who has a lot of sensory integration knowledge and can keep up with a 100-mile-a-minute boy." I thank the good Lord, who I believe moves everything around and brings the right people into your life at the right times, that this scheduler made the best choice for us. She put us with Mrs. Hannah Ragan, and she was the perfect fit for our needs.

While I waited for our OT sessions to begin, I did what only a trained behavioral interventionalist would do. I started a "behavioral logbook" of observations! My previous job as a therapist was to look at the ABCs of behavior: the antecedent (what happens before), the behavior (which is targeted to change) and the consequence (what happens after, positive or negative). The basic idea is that if you can figure out what is driving the negative behavior, you can increase or decrease it by changing the antecedents and consequences. To keep myself from going crazy with worry of the unknown, I dug in the only way I could — by analyzing his behavior. It made me feel useful and more in control. I charted the different behaviors I saw, how frequently they occurred, what time of day, how we reacted and finally whether the behavior increased or decreased in response. I couldn't make much sense of what I was charting, but I figured if I could put the information into his OT's hands, she would see patterns hidden in the data and know how to intervene.

I walked in to our first session with Mrs. Hannah and handed her the binder. She spent most of the time reading the observations while an intern played with Jacob in the sensory gym (a lovely padded space with different types of swings, a slide, ball pit, rock climbing wall and lots of toys). Then, a wonderful thing happened. For the first time since our story had begun, I felt like I had someone with the weapons needed stepping onto the battlefield with me. Everything Mrs. Hannah told me made sense regarding Jacob's wild and wooliness, and I finally felt my chest relax in relief. She knew how to move our family in a direction of progress and healing. I didn't have to do this alone.

Over time, I learned how critically important it was to move past the diagnosis and not get stuck in denial or self-pity. We needed to press on. We needed to do the hard work. The benefits would be worth it come reaping time.

Over time, I learned how critically important it was to move past the diagnosis and not get stuck in denial or self-pity. We needed to press on. We needed to do the hard work. The benefits would be worth it come reaping time.

These early days were hard in *so* many ways. I coped and pressed on plenty, but doing so isn't always easy. In fact, it rarely is. I remember breaking down in an embarrassing, snotty, ugly cry when one of my life-long friends came up after church and nonchalantly asked how life was going. Eric and I hadn't told many people about Jacob's diagnosis, all the doctor appointments or us starting therapy, but boy did she ever find out — whether she wanted to or not! The overwhelming grief and fear of it all suddenly welled up inside me, and my whole face contorted before I could put a lid on it. She hugged me tight as I told her bits and pieces of what we were going through. I knew she wasn't really understanding much of what I said, but I shared as much as my quivering mouth allowed and then pried myself loose to escape to the car. When I got in and closed the passenger side door Eric, just patted my leg. I finally took a breath, found my resolve and threw myself back into the action plan.

I'll also never forget the day I shut myself and Jacob in the dark walk-in closet at my in-laws' house, me releasing this gush of emotion while he self-regulated by rigidly rocking back and forth, repeating his catch phrase at the time to self-soothe. *Basketball, basketball, basketball.* The birthday party — with the paper flying, everyone talking and laughing, and him jumping, squealing, spinning and crashing — was too much stimulation for *both* of us. *Basketball, basketball, basketball.* We stayed hidden away until Eric got worried and came looking for us. I still remember his face when he peered in the door and said, "Honey, what are you all doing in the closet?" *Basketball, basketball, basketball.*

For me, having a special needs child means wrapping my mind around always finding ways to go the extra mile, constantly preparing for the unknown, explaining something a million times, and guarding myself against misunderstandings, disapproving comments and looks (sometimes from people I cared deeply about who just couldn't empathize). It is the hardest battle I've fought, but fighting through the mental and emotional parts to get to the intervention work has been a game-changer. I want you to hear me loud and clear: this experience can make you, your child and your family stronger and more resilient if you open your heart to the risk and build the right team to tackle it. Work toward progress, not perfection. Maximize the strengths. Minimize the weaknesses.

I want you to hear me loud and clear: this experience can make you, your child and your family stronger and more resilient if you open your heart to the risk and build the right team to tackle it.

Now that we are on the other side of Jacob's SPD diagnosis (for Jacob is now 10 years old and doing well physically, socially and academically) I can affirm early intervention made the difference. We did in fact *change* his nervous system functioning, and basically *healed* the disorder. Read on, my friend, and let hope bubble up.

WHAT DO I DO IF MY LOVED ONE IS DIAGNOSED WITH SPD AT AN OLDER AGE?

You just read this critical statement: *In most cases **early intervention** is a vital key in treating nervous system disorders. The nervous system is very malleable (or moldable) in the formative years, so the more changes you can make early on the better; it gets more difficult to change nervous system functioning as a person ages.*

You might be thinking you missed this magical window of time ... but that is just another shade of grief and denial designed to hold you back from helping your loved one reach their full potential, whatever that may be! Do not stop seeking answers and support. In fact, in the coming chapters you will discover therapies and interventions that could still be applied to your older child, teenager or even an adult! It has been proven that changes to the brain and nervous system can be made even into old age ... it just may *take longer and be harder work.*

You can improve your loved one's functioning one day at a time! Don't ever stop believing in the fierce power of love and dedication.

Hannah's Professional Opinion

Can you explain more about what sensory processing disorder (SPD) is and the different sub-types?

Sensory processing is the undertaking of the brain interpreting and organizing sensory experiences (touch, sound, smell, taste, sight, movement, body awareness, etc.). A simple explanation of sensory processing dysfunction is an impairment with the brain's ability to register the incoming sensory information accurately and respond with the appropriate actions. As with most disorders, the presentation of SPD can vary from one individual to the next. Individuals may demonstrate more or less hypersensitive (sensory-avoiding) or hyposensitive (sensory-seeking) responses in any given situation, because the sensory information is either overwhelming them or not enough to allow for typical functioning. Furthermore, the sensory and motor systems work simultaneously in order for the body to function properly. If one system is impaired it can often affect the other. This can present as coordination or motor planning difficulties due to possible deficits with the proprioceptive system, which is one's body awareness.

Why is it hard for families to suspect SPD on their own? What should you look for?

First of all, SPD is a diagnosis not commonly accepted or understood in the medical community, even though it is gaining more weight all the time. Whether this is due to lack of education or awareness of children with sensory difficulties, or a lack of research/evidence, I can't say for sure. I believe SPD is difficult to suspect because it is so little known among professionals and the general public. It is also a *hidden* disability. Children who present characteristics of SPD do so only in their behavior. They often do not "look different" or have any other medical equipment like crutches or wheelchairs to set them apart from their typical peers. People, therefore, judge them on their behavior and either think it is typical or a result of lack of discipline at home. When parents feel attacked by others' judgement, their natural reaction is to feel guilty and responsible themselves, and then ignore, control or hide the child's behaviors the best they can. However, I believe that instead of looking at behaviors only as something to stop or change, we need to look at them as an opportunity to learn about the child and understand the reasons *behind* their behavior. Behavior is often a reaction to a trigger of some sort and that the child has an immature form of communication or lack of coping skills to handle it appropriately. If we, as parents and professionals, can get to the root of the behaviors, we can teach the child to understand themselves and give them the intervention tools they need to meet their own needs. Then, they can cope better in family life and the community.

If you are a parent who suspects SPD as a diagnosis, some common behaviors you might observe include: difficulty in social situations, abnormal sleep patterns, delays with toilet training, difficulty in coordinating how to dress themselves or clothing may appear to agitate them, a very selective diet, and delays with communication skills.

Why is it important for families to pursue evaluations and treatment if they suspect SPD?

It is proven that early intervention is optimal for individuals diagnosed with SPD due to the brain's plasticity when we are young. Plasticity, or neuroplasticity, is the brain's ability to make changes. As we get older, the brain loses some of its plasticity. Hopefully, as science and research progress, we will be able to see concrete evidence, such as comparable images, of how early treatment changes the brain structure in children with SPD. It is my opinion that treatment must somehow create new, better functioning, or rerouted neuropathways because the range of behavioral changes I see in clients supports the understanding of how their nervous systems can process their senses more accurately than before treatment.

Professionals also have many available tools to enhance life's experiences, thus reducing a child's stress exponentially. If the child has differences in how they process the world around them, it is important for them to learn the individual needs of their own bodies and how best to address those needs. If a child can achieve self-awareness, I believe they will also achieve a healthier level of self-esteem, happiness and success in future life.

Can you briefly explain what happens during an evaluation?

Every facility has their own evaluation process. At the facility I work at, the occupational therapy evaluation is extensive and thorough. Initially, an intake form is sent to the parents/caregivers that includes demographic information, reason for referral and primary concerns so we can understand the client and their family's needs before meeting them. This is how the therapists are able to determine where they want to focus the initial session using their choice of various standardized and interview-based assessments.

There is not a specific or standardized process utilized once the evaluation starts, as every evaluating therapist has their own method, but in general, the therapist will focus on areas of concern and seek to learn more — and see firsthand — why the patient was referred.

They will watch the child for any signs of delays or deficits, and assessments may be given to the parent to fill out or to the child in the form of various activities and tasks. Discussion with the family is a big part of the evaluation. Their experience helps determine how the child performs in other environments. Occupational therapy takes on a holistic approach to evaluation and treatment in that therapists seek to look at the whole picture (areas of occupation, client factors — such as values, beliefs, spirituality — performance skills, performance patterns, context and environment, and activity demands) to determine underlining cause and/or where to begin with a treatment plan.

Why did Jacob behave the way he did in the evaluation?

From reviewing all the reports, I believe Jacob's system was on high alert because he was in a new, potentially unsafe and unexplored environment. That type of situation can completely overstimulate a child with SPD. These are all things we look for during the initial evaluation.

What about his behavior might a therapist recognize as SPD and not just an unruly child?

His inability to sit still, excessively looking in the mirror and hyper awareness of sounds that others usually tune out can all be signs of SPD. Having difficulty copying lines and shapes or working puzzles can be examples of deficits in fine motor skills and overall visual-motor processing. His use of excessive force on his pencil while writing shows modulation difficulties. Professionals are trained to tune into certain behaviors and distinguish these from others through clinical observation skills and various assessments.

Why is having a good client-therapist-parent fit so important? How do we go about switching if it is not?

Trust is paramount to success. Trust promotes good communication and follow through between child and therapist, as well as caregiver and therapist. The parent-therapist fit, in addition to the child-therapist fit, is important because often times if the parent is comfortable and trusting of the therapist then generally their child will be as well. If a parent does not feel comfortable with their therapist for any reason, it is critical that they talk to their therapist about it. If you are struggling in any way with the client-therapist-parent relationship, a few questions you might ask are:

1. Do you feel comfortable talking to your therapist about any concerns you have regarding your child?

2. Do you feel the therapist respects you as a parent?

3. Do you feel that therapist has your child's best interests at heart?

If you answered no to any of these questions, I would first try talking with your therapist since you may be experiencing a lack of communication. If you've tried to communicate your needs or concerns and still do not see the desired changes, then approach the facility's administration or scheduler and ask for another therapist. If they will not accommodate your request or you still do not get the desired results with a new therapist, then consider switching facilities. I cannot stress enough how important an open line of communication is between the parent and the therapist. When the relationship is not working, keep searching for the right fit for your family. It isn't anyone's fault, and it is a perfectly acceptable step to take on behalf of your child's best interest.

Why is it so important for families to accept their diagnosis and get ready to participate in whatever therapy is recommended?

This is a very difficult question, because every family has their own way of processing a diagnosis and getting in the mental and emotional place to participate in a treatment plan. Some families may get so wrapped up in the diagnosis that they become obsessed and put undue stress on themselves and the child. They may forget to take it slowly and remember they are good parents doing everything they possibly can. Other families may not be able to accept their reality at the time of diagnosis and fall into denial, not doing anything at that time. Still other families may have a bleak prognosis from birth and not want to put their child through any therapy at all.

You never know the outcome of a situation, and often life will surprise us. Every child is worth the fight, and their potential future is worth the effort. I don't see a lot of denial myself, because in general, by the time a client is referred to therapy the family has been looking for help and is ready to accept the diagnosis and the treatment program that follows.

For the best possible outcome, it is important for families to accept their child's diagnosis and participate in therapy. Research proves early intervention is the best way to offset deficits and make gains in a child's development. If a child begins therapy while they are young and still developing, we can assist in making them as functional as possible while they grow. If a child seeks therapy when they are older, often times they have already learned nonfunctional coping strategies and maladaptive behaviors to handle their body sensations. In these cases, we have a lot of work to "undo" all that learning and reteach functional and appropriate coping skills and behavior. Changes and improvement of life can definitely be made at later ages; it is just much easier for the child if we can circumvent the relearning process and teach them positive strategies first by having them begin therapy at younger ages.

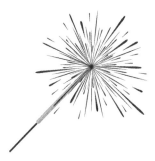

PART TWO

INTERVENTIONS THAT WORKED FOR US

Food Allergies

Biomedical Intervention

The Sensory Diet

Wilbarger Protocol

Integrative Listening Therapies

Astronaut Training

Visual Aids

The SPIO Suit

Environmental Adaptations

Brain Training

Interactive Metronome Training

The Crawling Program

ADHD Medications

Martial Arts

The Skinny on Cost and Time Commitments

Hannah's Professional Opinion

FOOD ALLERGIES

A lot of people want to know *why* their kid has sensory processing disorder (SPD). It is my opinion that genetics set the kid up on the cliff, and the environment tips him or her over the edge.

Through personal experience and engagement with other parents and professionals, I have learned that SPD (as well as other diagnoses such as autism, attention deficit or hyperactivity disorder — ADD/ADHD, asthma and allergies) is a three-pronged problem, and it's on the rise. The three parts include the interdependent nervous system, immune system and gastrointestinal system. Genetics play an important part in the functioning of these companion systems as does environment.

The nervous system, where you notice symptoms of SPD, is just the tip of the iceberg. Your neurons (and immunity) are affected by your gastrointestinal system — so that's a big hidden danger only found under the surface. If your gastrointestinal system is not working properly or is allergic to foods that you constantly bombard it with (most people don't even know they have food allergies), then not only will it cause nervous system malfunction, but your immune system will also go haywire as it can't keep up with all the allergens and environmental toxins bombarding it from every side! Your immune system can get stressed, causing you to frequently get sick or, because of the compromised immune system, children may not be able to tolerate vaccinations (especially at young ages).

Often times, the extended family members of a person with SPD are loaded with autoimmune disorders but people rarely connect these dots and understand why they are linked. I was diagnosed with Sjögren's syndrome after Jacob's diagnosis of SPD, and *then* realized there are myriad autoimmune disorders in our family tree. If you want to tackle SPD intervention head on, I urge you to look under the surface at the gastrointestinal and immune systems with biomedical intervention — as well as therapies for the nervous system.

I was diagnosed with Sjögren's syndrome after Jacob's diagnosis of SPD, and *then* realized there are myriad autoimmune disorders in our family tree.

I've always believed that nothing happens by chance, but my faith was deepened to new levels throughout my family's SPD journey. In fact, I believe that God led me to an early career in behavioral therapy to prepare me for Jacob's diagnosis. When I was hired for my first job in that profession, the company I worked for gave me two books to read, one of which is called *Unraveling the Mystery of Autism and Pervasive Developmental Disorder: A Mother's Story of Research & Recovery* by Karyn Seroussi. I know Jacob did not have autism, but sensory processing disorder accompanies people on the autism spectrum, from high-functioning ADHD and Asperger's syndrome to low-functioning, severe autism. I remember this book from my training, because it was all about the biological and immunological links between diet, autism and overall behavior. It was dense research to get through at the time because it wasn't relevant to me as a young adult, but for some reason I was still attached to it. It set on my bookcase gathering dust for almost nine *years.* When I found out my littlest one had a similar neurological disorder with behavioral implications, it was the first book I reached for. What pertinent information did my subconscious remember? Could Jacob have food allergies or sensitivities? Could a specialized diet help him calm down and think more clearly? I read it again with heightened interest, and I started to connect some really important dots.

The author reminded me that if gluten and casein proteins cannot be broken down properly, they can act as opiates in the brain, creating widespread havoc in the nervous system similar to hallucinogenic drugs. The sense organs can then be affected to the point that the brain cannot filter out what is important from what is not. This is how diet can affect behavior.

The author reminded me that if gluten and casein proteins cannot be broken down properly, they can act as opiates in the brain, creating widespread havoc in the nervous system similar to hallucinogenic drugs.

I believed Jacob's body processed the gluten and casein proteins ineffectively, which is why he seemed so disconnected from reality and in his own sensory world. We omitted gluten, casein and dye from his diet over the course of a year, but started seeing positive changes in mere days. The little boy who I had once backed against a wall, pleading with him to look at me and listen to my words while his eyes rapidly darted to the left and right and up and down while his body vibrated with energy, was suddenly calmer, more focused and aware of his surroundings. The best part is when he went from utilizing a few words to create choppy requests and responses (when we could get that out of him) to full-fledged, intelligent *sentences*. We didn't even know he had such language within him!

I first noticed these amazing changes one morning when he walked out of his bedroom with a stuffed racecar and said, "Mommy, this is Baby Lightening. He's my baby, and we have to take care of him. I will feed him, and you change his diaper. Change it like this." He showed me how he wanted me to make-believe with him. I cried for joy! First, Jacob never *walked* anywhere (he ran, jumped and bumped into things). Secondly, he had never played with a single toy! He would hold them, spin their wheels, throw them, use them in some way for his sensory fulfillment ... but he had never functionally *played* with them in the way they were intended. Here he was, not only carrying on a full conversation with me, but he had come up with a play scheme all by himself and wanted me to join in the fun!

So, why is gluten such a big deal for the nervous system? Why did taking it out of Jacob's diet make such a huge difference? One example highlighted in *Wheat Belly: Lose the Wheat, Lose the Weight, and Find Your Path Back to Health* by William Davis, MD, explains it well. Gluten proteins escape the intestines during digestion, get past the blood brain barrier and bond with the same receptors that *opiates* (like heroin and cocaine) bond with. They have actually used drugs like naloxone (which immediately brings down a "high" from illegal drugs) to counter the effects and block the receptors from bonding in people with sensory symptoms. Another experiment Davis's book highlighted was with people diagnosed with schizophrenia. The study noticed that when they did not consume gluten, their hallucinations diminished rapidly and consistently. Science has proven gluten negatively affects the brain and tampers with how we experience the world around us.

When we ditched the gluten protein in his diet, Jacob also slept better. He went from thrashing and crying in his sleep and waking four to five times a night to resting still and peaceful, with maybe only one waking. This was a *miracle*, people. As for the itchy, mealy rash that previously covered so much of his body, it became smooth and then disappeared.

Casein, the protein found in dairy products, was the next to go. Funny enough, when we omitted gluten from Jacob's diet, we saw a sudden spike in his desire for milk and cheese. I had read in Seroussi's book that this could happen. It helped me understand how gluten and casein are molecularly similar, so when you take one out of your diet you crave the other — like *drugs*. Jacob went from drinking one cup of milk a day to begging for four cups even during the night. We switched out our regular milk for a nut-based option, changed our butter to a vegan spread, and took away cheese, opting for a soy-based yogurt instead. With every step we took, his ability to think, reflect and communicate kept improving. I was still charting his problem behaviors in the behavior log binder at this time, along with what he ate and drank, and we could see the negative behavior tally marks falling steadily. He improved so drastically that I eventually forgot to write about his days in the binder at all! It sat on my kitchen counter collecting dust as we reclaimed little parts of a normal life. The gut-brain connection is a pivotal piece of understanding that can change so many lives.

The gut-brain connection is a pivotal piece of understanding that can change so many lives.

As a family, we supported Jacob's diet adjustments by also omitting gluten and casein and, together, we all experienced amazing results. Eric, Annabelle and I all started feeling better with the healthier food choices in the house. This change helped me realize I had food sensitivities my whole life without knowing it. I was the stereotypical sick "allergy kid" and had some gastrointestinal issues that persisted into adulthood. Go figure. Likewise, Annabelle always had stomach aches at night and had been quite an anxious kid. When she stopped consuming dairy, however, her stomach aches stopped completely, and her moods mellowed. Isn't it amazing how what you eat can impact how you feel?

The next step after removing gluten and casein from our diet was to add a probiotic to the good nutritional base. This helped heal Jacob's permeated gut the food sensitivities had caused, as well as restore the gastrointestinal balance and support a healthier immune system for both children. Like a chip off the old block, these two kids were also known as "allergy babies" before we cleaned up their diets. They suffered from sinus infections that turned into multiple ear infections or bronchitis a couple times a month, and the doctors kept increasing the antibiotic and steroid use. We owned a mini nebulizer machine for their breathing treatments and had a stock of Albuterol and Pulmicort to use at our discretion. Shortly before the SPD diagnosis and the drastic nutrition changes, we had actually started them on regular allergy shots. After we omitted gluten and casein, the sick visits stopped. We even discontinued the allergy shots, because their seasonal allergies improved, too! We didn't have to see a doctor for an illness for over a year, and then it was only once or twice a year after that. Let that sink in. That is how important and *healing* allergy-free nutrition can be.

About six months after making the diet changes, we decided to remove artificial food-dyes from our diets as well. Research linked artificial dyes to ADHD symptoms in many children, and it was my opinion that his struggles with attention, energy and impulsivity, even at the young age of 3, were headed down that path. I was going to leave no stone unturned regardless. Once again, we saw his behaviors decrease and his ability to process information and interact more appropriately increase!

People may scoff and say there is no connection between artificial dyes and behavior, but they weren't at the frozen yogurt shop when Jacob accidentally ingested them. Eric had taken him one day by himself but forgot to bring his naturally flavored gummy bears for the topping. (We always tried to take substitute foods and treats with us wherever we went.) Eric didn't realize the mistake and loaded him up with regular gummy bears from the toppings bar! In less than 10 minutes, Jacob was standing on his chair, flapping his arms and making incomprehensible noises like a squawking bird, and his yogurt dumped upside down on the floor. Eric quickly cleaned up the mess and carried the gooney bird to the car. If there had been any doubt about the effects of his diet intervention, it was forever solidified as absolute *truth* in our minds that day! The old adage is true: *you are what you eat.* If you fuel your body with clean, allergy-free foods, you will function at your best with a strong body and clear mind.

The old adage is true: *you are what you eat.* If you fuel your body with clean, allergy-free foods, you will function at your best with a strong body and clear mind.

Likewise, when Jacob got a hold of gluten or casein, we could identify the mistake right away. He would start in with violent stomach cramps that gave way to thrashing nightmares that kept us all up, followed by a few days of the vilest bowel movements you could imagine. Don't even try to picture it! It was *awful,* like the food was ripping up his insides as it moved through. Adults with gluten intolerance describe the feeling of similar episodes as knives moving through their intestinal tract. Jacob's behaviors would go back through the roof again as well, until his body worked it all out of his system and started to heal again. I firmly believe if we didn't get the diet in place early on that the occupational therapy gains wouldn't have been nearly as effective. This was block one, the springboard for all subsequent healing.

I urge you to learn about different food allergies. Your child might be allergic to soy, nuts, corn, night-shade vegetables ... there are many that seem to exacerbate the symptoms of autism, ADHD and SPD. Get the proper tests and rule it in or rule it out. What's it going to hurt?

BIOMEDICAL INTERVENTION

An allergy-free diet is the first building block for repairing nervous system malfunction. The second building block is the broader branch of medicine known as biomedical intervention. Most importantly for our family, this next-step intervention included detoxification measures and customized supplementation that proved beneficial on so many accounts.

There came a time after talking with other parents who had kids with sensory processing disorder (SPD), researching on my own, and watching Jacob carefully, that I felt alone. It appeared that I was the only one bringing new ideas to the physician-parent-patient table regarding this important topic for our family. A friend who worked in the medical field reminded me that most doctors are not trained in the kind of proactive, preventative medicine I was seeking for Jacob. They are trained to react, to treat illness and disorders after you're sick … not to prevent. I wanted to have a "medical home" that knew more about healing the body from the *inside out*. So, I began the tedious search for doctors, both a new pediatrician and an integrationist (or naturopathic) who could better support our family.

It appeared that I was the only one bringing new ideas to the physician-parent-patient table regarding this important topic for our family.

I finally found a pediatrician that not only was a good fit for our family, but was willing to work with an integrationist. I was most excited about a book recommendation he gave me. *Healing the New Childhood Epidemics: Autism, ADHD, Asthma, and Allergies: The Groundbreaking Program for the 4-A Disorders* was co-written by Dr. Kenneth Bock, a New York doctor who worked with a group of DAN (Defeat Autism Now) doctors, and Cameron Stauth. Dr. Bock had researched and created a biomedical approach to healing these major neurological and immunological disorders that seem to be extremely prevalent in our day and age.

I took the book with me everywhere I went, devouring its research-dense pages. It opened up so much understanding into Jacob's diagnosis and why today's American children seem to be getting more and more sick. Dr. Bock supports with research that "genetics loads the gun and environment pulls the trigger" with these 4-A epidemics. You cannot help the genetics you inherit, but so many people do not realize how their environment can impact their genetics (such as toxins like vaccines, processed or genetically modified food, air pollution, etc.).

The more pages I read, the more I noticed that Jacob had so many commonalities with the children highlighted in Dr. Bock's book including: family history of autoimmunity, exposure to toxins in utero (I was vaccinated with the swine flu vaccine when pregnant, not to mention the chemicals in the foods I unknowingly ate), accelerated vaccine schedule because of missed doses when he was an infant, chronic sinus/ear infections that led to two sets of ear tubes, multiple rounds of antibiotics/steroids ... the similarities continued on and on. The bottom line was that Jacob was a more *genetically fragile* child that we didn't know about soon enough, and his interaction with too many environmental factors helped to pull the trigger on his nervous system malfunction. Dr. Bock mentioned in his book that autism, Asperger's syndrome, pervasive developmental disorder-not otherwise specified (PDD-NOS), SPD, ADHD and even mild learning disabilities like dyslexia are all on the same sliding continuum of nervous system function. What you get "labeled" with notes where you are on that scale, diagnosed by the kind of symptoms you have, their intensity and frequency.

If environment cripples the immune, gastrointestinal and nervous systems, it stands to reason that we should be able to correct the imbalances by altering diet, supplementing deficient nutrients and helping the body detoxify the metals and toxins that are causing the damage.

If environment cripples the immune, gastrointestinal and nervous systems, it stands to reason that we should be able to correct the imbalances by altering diet, supplementing deficient nutrients and helping the body detoxify the metals and toxins that are causing the damage.

My eyes were opened further to how if Jacob's neurological and behavioral problems were directly linked to his biology, there were steps we could take to get his body back in line with how God designed it to be. From that point on, I became focused on getting his vitamin, nutrient and antioxidant levels checked regularly for excesses or deficiencies.

A friend in our local SPD support group recommended an integrationist who provided this type of review. Armed with my Dr. Bock book and a list of interventions we had done through occupational therapy (OT) and diet thus far, we went to meet him. Jacob had been getting OT for nearly a year, so I knew that a packed backpack of sensory intervention toys would help keep him calm and busy during the visit. You remember how he behaved at the OT evaluation, right? I was determined to not repeat *that* experience.

SPD wasn't playing by the rules that day, however. No matter what sensory intervention strategy I pulled out, Jacob morphed into the old fully-loaded Captain Destructo upon walking into the office. He literally tried to climb the walls ... physically tried to scale them, I tell you. Then, once he made it as far up as his body and strength would allow, he slid back down like a slug with no suction cups. When that game was no longer stimulating him, he crawled under the chairs like they were a tunnel and kicked and threw the blocks in the play corner, all while I tried to check in, fill out paper work and corral him in between the front desk and my legs. That's when I could catch him.

Thankfully Eric arrived just in time to help out, but things only escalated once we got into the little exam room with the doctor. Jacob had a wild look in his eyes — hyper, anxious and fearful all at the same time — and he never stopped *moving*. For two hours he didn't stop. He was on the table, off the table, lay on the table, slide off the table, run to the door, bang on the door, climb onto the windowsill, climb back down, pull out his toys, throw his toys, blow bubbles in the doctor's face, cram snacks in his mouth, dribble snacks out of his mouth, try to touch the doctor's computer, spin in circles, jump up and down, bang on anything and everything, and every once in a while he would let out this war-whoop of a high-pitched squeal while shaking his head AND banging on something! Are you tired after reading that? It was worse living it. We tried everything to calm him down including taking turns applying deep pressure by squeezing on him, but my hair was too tickly on his face and Eric's whiskers were too scratchy. Off came the shoes and socks, which was one of Jacob's tell-tale signs of complete sensory overload and ensuing meltdown. Remember that sliding scale of nervous system dysfunction? If this was your only experience with Jacob, you would have thought he was *severely* autistic.

Eric and I were truly mentally, physically and emotionally exhausted by the time we left the office. Even though our nerves were shot, the silver lining was that the doctor got a very good look at Jacob in full force. Poor Jacob was spent, too. This incident was not a discipline issue or even a lack of sensory diet issue. We had done everything by the book. This was true SPD when all of the sensory information jammed up in his brain from the new smells, sights, lights, movement, change in routine, new experience and probably from empathizing with the stress and anxiety from Eric and me as well. He could not process or function through his brain's traffic jam. I felt so sorry for him — to look into the scared, desperate eyes of your child, seeing his soul trapped inside an unruly, pulsating body of adrenaline and confusion is truly painful for the parent as well.

He calmed down once we got back into the car, grateful to be back in our own space with the familiar smells, absence of people and decreased stress. The intense SPD reactions switched off as quickly as they had flared. He started carrying on full conversations like nothing had happened. He behavior was like night and day. He looked a little sheepish at me in the rear-view mirror, like he knew he had been "bad," so I took the opportunity to tell him how much I loved him and that I knew he really tried hard to keep his engine just right in the office. I told him I knew his engine was running high, and I was glad it was coming back down now. Then I asked him how it felt to be in that doctor's office, expecting his usual answer of "fireworks inside me." He whispered, "fire in my face." His self-expression conjured a picture in my mind of him playing with a sparkler on the Fourth of July. The fiery end got too close and Jacob felt the the pop and sizzle, but no matter what he did to scramble away, the sparkler of SPD was held to his body — the explosive intensity burning his tender face.

He crashed on the way home and slept for *three* hours. His engine, understandably, had run out of gas.

Then I asked him how it felt to be in that doctor's office, expecting his usual answer of "fireworks inside me." He whispered, "fire in my face."

At the follow-up appointment the doctor agreed that Jacob's nervous system was most definitely inflamed and that was putting it nicely. He recommended starting the biomedical intervention with some baseline tests such as blood, urine and stool that would tell us how his body was currently working, and we would move forward with aligning his biology from there.

When the testing results came back in, we discovered he had an opportunistic bacterium called Achromobacter in his gut (as opposed to pathogenic or the kind that actively makes you sick). This was responsible for the disruption of digestion, absorption, nutrient production, pH and immune states. The most surprising find, however, was that out of 16 key antioxidants, vitamins and minerals, only two were within normal range; eight were borderline deficient and six were highly deficient! With this newfound knowledge, we set up a customized vitamin regimen to help adjust his levels back into efficient ranges, especially supporting the B-vitamins that are so important to nervous system function. We gave this plan a year to work and repeated the blood and urine tests and added genomic testing the next year to see the progress that was made, and it was astounding. Where he had been deficient in 14 out of 16 major antioxidants, vitamins and minerals, one year of specific supplementation had cut it in *half*. He was deficient in only five and in high need of just two! The ones he continues to be persistently deficient in is alpha-lipoic acid (for brain health) and B-12 (for nervous system health).

The genomic testing both confirmed his gluten allergy and revealed
that he has trouble processing sulfurs and environmental toxins.
Usually a person's methylation process, a chemical reaction in
every cell and tissue of the body that helps detoxify the body of
harmful toxins, would "clean up" this problem. Jacob's methylation
process, however, is impaired. The integrationist likened his detox
challenges to pouring honey through a funnel. It will go through
eventually, but it is slow and backs up easily ... and where does
detox sludge spill into? It overflows into the *nervous system* — thus
impacting brain function and sensory integration. With this new
information we turned our attention to cleaning up our environment,
which was overloading Jacob's body with toxins, the same way we
cleaned up our diet. This was an undertaking that took about two
years. You wouldn't believe how many non-food household items
contain gluten and dyes, not to mention other harmful chemicals!
We switched to the most natural, allergy-friendly ingredients for the
following products: laundry detergent, fabric softener, dryer sheets,
shampoo, body wash, lotion, sunscreen, toothpaste, mouthwash and
cleaning supplies. While it was overwhelming initially as we considered the lifestyle changes we needed to make, we took it a little at
a time, knowing that it would make a positive difference. And it has!

**While it was overwhelming initially as we considered
the lifestyle changes we needed to make, we took it
a little at a time, knowing that it would make a positive
difference. And it has!**

HEALTHY LIVING IS CLEAN LIVING

There are a lot of ways to clean up the environment you live in every day, from what you clean your house with to what goes on your skin and hair. For most of my cleaning I use chemical-free Norwex products and water because that was what was well-known at the time we were making changes. Now there are even more "clean" options out there to choose from, including Meliora products, The Honest Company and Arbonne.

For those interested in what my household uses daily, here's some of my favorites!

- My Norwex products for house cleaning include: microfiber, self-cleansing envirocloths; kitchen, window cloths; veggie and fruit scrub cloth; cleaning paste; dusting mitt; microfiber superior mop with wet/dry reusable pads and rubber brush; bathroom cleaner and spirinett scrubbers.

- For bathing and washing clothes, we found a friend who makes basic allergy-free laundry soap powder and coconut oil soap for us! We also have Norwex body cloths and coconut based shampoo/conditioner. When we goof up and don't use these products, Jacob's mealy skin rash comes back overnight.

- Just for us girls ... Annabelle and I use Physician's Formula make-up (remember, I have an autoimmune disorder so if I put something on my skin that sets off my inflammation response, my eyes will swell shut), and we cleanse our faces with Arbonne products.

Changing the cleaning and personal products we use was life-changing for everyone in our family, including Jacob. Once, when we had stayed late at my parents' house, I bathed Jacob there so he'd be ready for bed in case he fell asleep in the car on the way home. I used regular shampoo and soap for him, and after drying off with towels that had been washed in a typical detergent, he wore one of Papaw's shirts on the ride home. One quick bath with everyday shampoo and detergent can't hurt, right? Wrong. In addition to a fresh rash, he was an overly sensitive bear to handle the next day. The toothpaste was too stingy. His clothes didn't feel right. He couldn't sit still at lunch. He was orally fixated as well, needing a lot of cold, crunchy ice in between blowing raspberries. I dragged him to a playground where he could run, jump and climb thinking that would give him the proprioceptive and vestibular input needed to regulate, but no matter what intervention I tried, he could not get his engine just right. After a warm Epsom salt bath (Epsom salts contain magnesium which binds with sugar molecules and can help decrease hyperactivity symptoms through the detoxification process, as well as being a natural stress reliever by boosting serotonin levels which gives a feeling of well-being and relaxation), and a nice rub down (deep pressure), he still laid awake for two and a half hours, wiggling and talking to himself. As if that wasn't rough enough, he had a bellyache all night and finally a cleansing, but messy, bowel movement in the morning (tell-tale signs he got a hold of an allergen).

When talking SPD, we found out firsthand just how important it is to evaluate your environment in addition to nutrition and supplementation. Chemicals in everyday products are proven neurotoxins that are put directly on your skin and get absorbed right into your blood circulation. The opportunity of being ingested and going through the lymphatic system first (which would help clean out some of the allergens and toxins before absorption) is a lost benefit.

Addressing Jacob's health from a biological standpoint laid the groundwork for OT to do their best work — and it helped the gains to stick. If your family is impacted with SPD, do your research and learn how biomedical interventions could apply to your child (keep in mind that not all SPD children have the same allergies and biological deficiencies), and find knowledgeable professionals (and eco-friendly businesses) to start your journey off on the healthiest foot possible. I *promise* you it is not a waste of time or money.

TO VACCINATE OR NOT TO VACCINATE? THAT'S AN IMPORTANT QUESTION.

This will always be a controversial topic, and I assure you I see both sides. Educate yourself well and talk with a trusted healthcare professional before you put anything into your own body or your child's. Many kids get vaccines daily and are *completely* fine! However, there is research that proves that vaccinations can be one of the environmental triggers that impacts nervous system malfunction. Thimerosal, which isn't in all vaccines, is pretty dangerous stuff. I take great pause with Jacob, because he is medically fragile in the sense of him having compromised immune and detox systems. I want him to be protected from these horrible diseases, but I also want to keep his nervous system healthy. I hope one day there will be some sort of middle ground in this great debate. Maybe the medical field can develop a way to screen out medically fragile children who are at risk of negative vaccine reactions and find ways to protect their health in all facets.

When vaccinating medically fragile children, here are some helpful tips I've learned through my research:

1. Postpone vaccinations if your child has been sick, is ill or you suspect is coming down with something (the immune system is already compromised at that point).

2. Give your child vitamin supplements before and after the vaccination to boost the immune system before it takes a hit.

3. Ask for single-dose vials and administer them one at a time over several weeks or months to give the body time to absorb, react and detox in between doses.

4. Give your child extra rest, fluids, and a healthy diet to boost the immune system.

5. If you have major concerns, especially with newborns and young children but still want to vaccinate, perhaps you can wait until your child is older with a more mature immune system.

If you are interested in learning more about how vaccinations can contribute to nervous system dysfunction or how to more safely administer them to medically fragile children, check out the book *Healing the New Childhood Epidemics: Autism, ADHD, Asthma, and Allergies: The Groundbreaking Program for the 4-A Disorders* co-written by Dr. Kenneth Bock, a New York doctor who worked with a group of DAN (Defeat Autism Now) doctors, and Cameron Stauth. Many pediatricians are open to alternate vaccination schedules if parents ask.

THE SENSORY DIET

While occupational therapy (OT) cannot fix the underlying issues of the gastrointestinal and immune systems, it does offer an excellent way to reduce sensory processing disorder (SPD) symptoms, gain age-appropriate skills that haven't been acquired thus far, and aid in nervous system healing. OT is key to gaining proper and customized knowledge in regard to how a body works, what it needs and how to help your loved one in their daily life at home and in the community.

When we met Mrs. Hannah, she likened Jacob to a "sensory bull-dozer." Quickly she was able to paint a very accurate picture of our experience at home. From the time Jacob could scoot across the floor, he craved stimulation — nothing else was relevant. I now understand that he bulldozed through experiences for the sensory input, never stopping to appreciate or learn from them. Every move he made was focused on feeding this bottomless pit of a monstrous nervous system.

During our first OT session, Hannah empowered us with information about "sensory diets" (coined by Occupational Therapist Patricia Wilbarger). While it may initially seem like a foreign concept, in reality it's very similar to how a nutritional diet feeds your body at different intervals throughout the day, warding off "hangry" reactions. Similarly, a sensory diet provides for the sensory needs of a child by both spreading out sensory input through the day and providing opportunities to take breaks from stimulation. This dependent, steady input helps a struggling child stay focused and engaged by organizing a nervous system that constantly misfires on its own.

A sensory diet is a personalized activity plan that needs to be designed by a professional, who has a working knowledge of the nervous system and how to satiate the child's needs without overwhelming the child. In Jacob's case, parts of his nervous system were dominantly dull even though at times he could be hypersensitive to incoming stimuli (remember, people with SPD can be both sensory seekers and sensory avoiders at different times). Generally, he was a sensory seeker with problems in impulsivity and body awareness. Where neurologically typical people get filled up with everyday activities to function appropriately, Jacob needed so much *more* to get the same sense of regulation.

A sensory diet is a personalized activity plan that needs to be designed by a professional, who has a working knowledge of the nervous system and how to satiate the child's needs without overwhelming the child.

A sensory diet comes in handy because you figure out what your child needs to stay regulated and sprinkle those appropriate activities throughout the day before the kid seeks out his needs in unhealthy, dangerous or inappropriate ways. For Jacob, this meant a steady diet of proprioceptive (a sensation caused when one joint impacts another, usually achieved through weight bearing activities such as push-ups, crawling, stomping, carrying, lifting, pushing, pulling, etc.) and vestibular input (the movement sense, like swinging, falling, spinning, etc.). These two more elusive senses work in tandem to provide your body with important information, like where your body is in space and relation to other people and objects. If Jacob's nervous system was dull and his brain was not correctly processing these senses, this likely explained why he was always forcefully colliding with people and the world around him. We told Jacob these new activities were his "heavy work" and "deep pressure" (sometimes we called the latter "snug as a bug" activities), and with my binder of home observations, we figured that he needed to be *fed* every two hours or so. Like pulling gluten out of the diet, when we put purposeful sensory activities in, we saw immediate results. His needs became more manageable over the course of a year, so we began to stretch sensory activities and intervention from every two hours to just a couple of times a day.

We often used several two-liter bottles filled with water to create various games involving lots of heavy lifting for the much-needed proprioceptive input. We played hide-and-seek, where he had to find the bottles and carry them back to his big storage bucket. We bowled with them as our pins using a weighted eight-pound exercise ball. We also made up pretend games that involved him having to move them around the house to rescue various family members from impending peril. We'd cry, "Super Jacob to the rescue!" and sometimes he would pick up two bottles at a time to aid the damsel in distress! What began as a critical component to Jacob's sensory diet soon became something that was fun for the whole family.

What began as a critical component to Jacob's sensory diet soon became something that was fun for the whole family.

Another successful strategy we used to feed his senses throughout the day was a crash pad we made out of pillows and blankets. Both of my kids would jump onto it and crawl over it (crawling on hands and knees is great proprioceptive input and crawling over an uneven surface adds to the benefit because it is challenging the core muscles). Occasionally, we would put puzzle pieces on one end of the pad and the puzzle tray on the other. Jacob would then crawl back and forth to get a piece several times in order to complete the puzzle. This approach also worked his fine motor needs with the manipulation of the interlocking puzzle pieces.

Wheelbarrow walking was one of our early favorites, too. After a year of mini strength-training, Jacob could actually wheelbarrow down the hall — down four steps, out the back door and then up into the car – with upper body strength alone. We knew we were raising a man, but we had no clue we were raising a muscle man!

For deep pressure (also proprioceptive input) we created a game called, "sack of taters." Jacob would sit in the center of a fleece blanket and we would pull up all four corners, cocooning him inside. Then we would throw him over our backs like a sack of taters and walk around the house with him. Not only did his body pushing against the tight blanket provide great pressure, but the gentle swaying motion of walking was added vestibular input that helped calm him. He could go into his sack of taters completely disorganized and over-stimulated and come out calm and thoughtful in a matter of *minutes*. This is the power of a good sensory diet.

He could go into his sack of taters completely disorganized and overstimulated and come out calm and thoughtful in a matter of *minutes*. This is the power of a good sensory diet.

To save our backs as he grew, however, we invested in buying a cocoon-style canvas swing that could hang from the ceiling of his room. Before Jacob began OT, he had no sense of getting dizzy. He could spin for a long time before he got his fill of vestibular input, so of course he loved the "spinny swing." He loved it so much, in fact, that he occasionally fell asleep inside from the calming sensation it gave him. We also bought a small trampoline for indoor use. I can't say enough about the benefits of jumping for a kid with SPD ... especially if it allows them to also fly off onto a crash pad! Vestibular plus proprioceptive input was the winning combo for our sensory-seeking boy.

For us, the sensory diet really provided a way to give Jacob what he needed to succeed and we found ways to fit the activities into our life naturally. He would help drag big garbage bags from the kitchen to the outside garbage can, switch wet heavy clothes from the washer to the dryer, and assist his Daddy in the family garden and yard work (his favorite way to help and satiate his needs)! When we went to the grocery, he would get heavy items off the bottom shelves, lift them in and out of the cart as needed, push the cart and help place our selections on the conveyor belt to check out. All of this input filled up his sensory bucket and helped him stay focused, engaged and organized. He could also feel *proud* he was making a positive contribution to the family.

The needs of your child may be different, which is why you should seek an evaluation with an occupational therapist who will be able to tell you what activities will best help your child stay regulated without accidentally over-stimulating him or her. Keep in mind, too, that the needs of each individual can also change over time. We went through a phase when proprioceptive and vestibular input was not resetting Jacob's nervous system like it previously had. He started chewing on his hands to a point where sometimes he gagging himself if he got too much of his fist in his mouth. He chewed his hands so much they started to chap, crack open and bleed! We had already purchased a "chewelry" necklace for such a need, but he refused it. So, I texted our therapist with a panicked call for help. (Yes, I had her personal phone number and was told to contact her when I needed to.) I cannot stress enough the importance of finding a knowledgeable therapist who is invested in the well-being of your family! She explained that SPD kids self-regulate in all different ways, and that Jacob was craving oral input to organize and calm his nervous system at this specific time in his development. She suggested letting him suck up apple-sauce or yogurt through a straw to work his mouth muscles and to think about incorporating cold, hard, crunchy, chewy or sour foods into his diet as each were "heavy work" for the mouth specifically, rather than the whole body. It was genius. The more I figured out how to give Jacob what he needed in an appropriate way, the less he sought it out in an inappropriate way — like chewing his hands down to nubs!

The more I figured out how to give Jacob what he needed in an appropriate way, the less he sought it out in an inappropriate way — like chewing his hands down to nubs!

After about a year of occupational therapy, Jacob's sensory needs shifted yet again. By this time, he had learned to recognize his needs and could ask for whatever input he was craving in order to self-regulate. He started responding to warm showers as a way to calm the nervous system, and it didn't matter if he wasn't dirty. If he woke up on a preschool morning and nervously asked to get in the shower, we happily turned on the water and let him run around in the spray for a few minutes. One time I peeked in, and he was lying in the tub on his back, holding his feet up to the sky so the spray would massage the soles of his feet! The amount of time it took to accommo-date his needs was *nothing* compared to surviving a high engine day in the absence of purposeful intervention. Likewise, if we had a really long day with a lot of stimulation, we would put him in the warm shower and let the beads of pounding water massage his stress away. He would then follow up with an Epsom salt bath. Afterward, he would emerge from all of these activities (when they were in season with his needs) a much calmer, happier and well-centered boy. My husband and I felt like detectives many days, on the hunt to figure out what sensory diet activities Jacob needed to regulate at which times. Then we taught *him* to recognize that feeling within and voice it to make our jobs easier.

The amount of time it took to accommodate his needs was *nothing* compared to surviving a high engine day in the absence of purposeful intervention.

Understanding my child came with a sense of euphoria. I finally understood his needs, what he was craving, and most importantly how to fulfill them so he didn't seek it out in negative or dangerous ways. I finally saw him for who he was and continue to see him for who he is. Most importantly, everyone involved was working as a team to modify the preconceptions of there being one right way to raise a child. I've come to learn that there are many ways!

Understanding my child came with a sense of euphoria.

Jacob is such a *sensational* kid in every aspect of the word. As my knowledge and "toolbox" of interventions grew in those early years, that greatness shined through the cracks of this disorder. I was determined to break it wide open before it was all said and done.

WILBARGER PROTOCOL

The Wilbarger Protocol (referred to as brushing therapy) was also developed by Patricia Wilbarger and became an important extension of our sensory diet. This protocol involved firmly brushing Jacob's body with a small surgical brush every two hours while he was awake and then follow-up with joint compressions. Mrs. Hannah showed us exactly how to brush him as we quickly learned that there was an order of body parts to brush in a specific way — from his arms down to his feet — while other body parts like the face, chest and stomach were to be avoided because of tactile sensitivity. She also gave us directions on the joint compressions. For that, we targeted his shoulders, elbows, wrists, hips, knees and ankles for 10 seconds each. As his system regulated through therapy and stayed regulated for longer periods of time, we slowly started spacing out his brushings and joint compressions until it ended up phasing out completely. While this brushing protocol is usually recommended for sensory avoiders (kids that are hyper-sensitive to stimuli) because it helps desensitize their bodies a little at a time which improves overall coping skills, it is also an awesome addition for sensory seekers.

The brushing therapy was like a mini deep pressure massage! If I stuck to the schedule and gave his sensory system the stimulation it needed to regulate at regular intervals, I saw the benefits immediately. He was able to better transition between daily activities.

He stayed calm for longer periods of time, and it improved his attention span.

What I loved most about this particular sensory intervention was that it was fast — fast to administer and fast to help. It was also quiet. For instance, church services were quite difficult for us to get through when he was young and in the height of his sensory processing disorder (SPD) struggles. Our children had always sat with us during services, and no matter what variety of snacks or little sensory toys we brought, they continued to fail at helping him sit through it. Before we knew about the Wilbarger Protocol, my mom and I would sandwich him between us and he would flip from putting his head in my lap and his feet in hers, to his head in hers and his feet in mine. He would hang off the bench, sometimes upside down, and eventually slide off the bench into the floor, where he would continue to squirm until the final Amen ended his pain. I was so self-conscious as a parent and embarrassed that I couldn't get control of my son, but what could I do? Remember, typical punishments only made his behavior worse, and missing church services was not an option for my family. So, we tried to make him "be good," but no matter how hard we tried, it continued to be ineffective. That's when the Wilbarger Protocol answered our prayers. It provided us with a tool that we could do in church, quickly and quietly, to give his body the stimulation it craved while calming and relaxing his anxiety at the same time. Church was full of his triggers — increase in people, noise and movement. Even when his next brushing wasn't due for another hour, if his engine started idling high out the brush would come. My mom and I would pass it between us — doing arms, hands, back, legs and feet (depending on whose lap his head and feet were in at the time), and then we would compress joints while we listened to the service. This effective strategy was another game-changer!

INTEGRATIVE LISTENING THERAPIES

The more we came to understand sensory processing disorder (SPD), the more we embraced how nutritional diet, biomedical intervention and the sensory diet interventions majorly contributed to success in winning this war. Smooth sailing, right? Buckle your seat belts, because the next sections dig deeper into the nitty-gritty details of how we saved our kid from SPD ... and, like most journeys, it often gets bumpy before it smooths out again.

Integrative listening therapies were Mrs. Hannah's next tool for recovery. These specialized music programs had headphones designed to play modulated music to stimulate the brain and help integrate the senses while improving nervous system function. If you think about it, music stimulates nearly every region of the brain and nearly every neural subsystem. Each brain lobe processes different aspects of the music, such as pitch, tempo, timbre, rhythm, lyrics ... the latter dividing further into not only sound recognition, but understanding the language, meaning, humor, sarcasm and more. Then those lobes, analyzing their own bits of music separately, have to communicate with each other and integrate a coherent picture of what we are hearing and feeling. No wonder it works so well to heal nervous system dysfunction! We did two of these programs, a basic one and an advanced one that added a bone conduction component to yield even higher results. Keep in mind that Jacob's senses were sending messages to his brain, but for whatever reason, the brain was not receiving them, processing them correctly or outputting the appropriate response 90% of the time. Mrs. Hannah proved this fact when she laid Jacob on the floor in certain positions and told him to move this or that limb. He couldn't do it. The brain-body disconnect was *real*.

Integrative listening therapies work on neuroplasticity, which is the rerouting and creating of new neural pathways in the brain. Jacob's brain basically went from a country road where few sensory messages and appropriate output behaviors traveled to a bustling highway where all things were possible. Sounds great, right? It *was* in the long run ... but day to day was tough work! We were focused on integrating the seven major senses so they would interact with each other the correct way, thus giving Jacob's brain information it needed to make good mental and behavioral decisions. While we knew the end goal, for a while it seemed like Jacob just fell apart.

Jacob's brain basically went from a country road where few sensory messages and appropriate output behaviors traveled to a bustling highway where all things were possible.

The proprioceptive and vestibular needs were being managed through the sensory diet, but shortly after starting integrative listening therapies Jacob's other senses went nuts. Unexpectedly we were dealing with biting, spitting and us saying phrases such as, "Jacob! Don't lick that!" He wanted to experience everything with his mouth. (You cringed, right?) When he wanted to talk to us in the car, we had to roll all the windows up, turn the radio off and be completely silent. He would get incredibly frustrated when he couldn't tune out the background noise long enough to get his words out, and often by the time we rushed to make the needed modifications he would have spiraled into full-blown meltdown because he forgot what he wanted to say. Bright lights started to bother him. The same boy who used to look into a flashlight and not understand why we rushed to pull it away now struggled in the opposite direction. The weirdest development was when he started to crave the smell of fish food. He would try to scale the dresser for just one sniff. Mrs. Hannah assured me that this temporary disorganization of his sensory system would lead to a higher-level organization by the end. I had to go fully on trust because every indicator looked otherwise. But his behavior change was a sign the therapy was *working*. He was finally processing sensory information that had never been processed before!

Everything about integrated listening therapy was grueling hard work. Have you ever considered how to keep a pair of bulky headphones (especially the second set, which was vibrating his skull through bone conduction) on a kid an hour a day for five days a week? Not that I was counting but that was 60 times total over a course of three months! I hope you never have to try. In addition to just getting him to merely *wear* them, there were sensorimotor activities to go with it. Whew!

The first 20 minutes of an integrated listening therapy session was devoted to sensorimotor activities such as balancing on a balance board, drawing large figure 8s across his midline, and touching his thumb to every fingertip. These exercises essentially got his sensory and motor systems talking to each other. He despised every minute of it. The second 20 minutes we spent jumping on the trampoline and throwing a ball (to expend some of that pent-up energy and frustration from the difficult activities while working on gross motor skills). Then, finally, the last 20 minutes incorporated sensory fun time with something hands-on, such as painting or playing with Play-Doh or shaving cream, to work on fine motor skills.

The first month utilizing this therapy approach dealt with integration and modulation of the senses. The second month targeted his core and praxis (when the two sides of your body move together, like catching a ball or crossing your midline to pick things up). The final phase, the third month, helped his communication centers in the brain. There were days I wanted to quit. Seriously. Jacob wanted to quit every day! But Mrs. Hannah gave me a beautiful analogy that has always stuck with me. It's like putting together a puzzle. It looks neat in the box, but to see the cohesive picture you have to dump out all the pieces, sort and organize them, and then put them together. When you first dump them out, it's overwhelming chaos. But, as it comes back together, you can see the picture emerge ... and when it's finished, it is *marvelous*.

It's like putting together a puzzle. It looks neat in the box, but to see the cohesive picture you have to dump out all the pieces, sort and organize them, and then put them together. When you first dump them out, it's overwhelming chaos. But, as it comes back together, you can see the picture emerge ... and when it's finished, it is *marvelous*.

Mrs. Hannah was right. Once we started to organize Jacob's "pieces," we started to see just how amazing the listening therapies were as they changed his brain function altogether. Before therapy Jacob didn't feel pain or temperature correctly, and he didn't have a sense of dizziness. For years I never needed to comfort him much when he got hurt. Once as a baby, he had a full-blown double ear infection that warranted an immediate steroid shot at the doctor's office. The doctor looked at me in amazement and said, "I don't know why this kid isn't screaming his head off." When he was 2 years old, he took a nosedive off my neighbor's porch and cut his hand open in the tender flesh between his pinkie and ring finger. He didn't shed a single tear then either. Instead, he just looked at his wound with four stitches with interest.

Before his diagnosis we didn't give any of this much thought. We chalked it up to him having a high threshold for pain. We never considered he wasn't *feeling* pain. His body was hurting, but the messages were not getting through to that little jam-packed brain of his! It was a dangerous, blissful state of ignorance. Throughout the listening therapy process we got to see him slowly process pain. He no longer immediately jumped up after a fall to keep running. He now got the message that he was hurt, and he would pause to look for the boo-boo. It was a muddy message from his nervous system, though. It alerted him just enough that something had happened but didn't give him enough info to actually figure out *where* he was scraped or bruised. Once he fell off his bike and skinned up his knee, blood dripped down his leg. He got up, said a delayed, "Ouch..." and looked at his arms. He checked out his hands, his elbows and his shoulders, and then looked very confused that he didn't see the offending body part. Annabelle ran up and pointed to his knee saying, "Oh, no, Bubby! You're bleeding!" He looked at the opposite knee, and then the ankle, and then the toes. I had to physically *touch* the side of the bleeding knee for him to finally see his gouged wound.

Jacob also did not feel temperatures correctly before we did integrative listening therapies. Warm bath water felt way too hot, and we would have to either run it considerably on the cold side or let the bath water sit for 15 minutes before he'd put a toe in to check for himself. He would also run outside barefoot in the snow before we could catch him since his brain would not process the message that his feet were freezing, literally! This is a great reminder of how SPD can be dangerous if not treated. During the second integrative listening program, the one that included bone conduction, Jacob's temperature glitch worked itself out. I remember the day in the tub when he jerked away from my hand and squealed, "Your hand is cold!" I was shocked and didn't know what happened at first. Then I called Eric into the bathroom and we celebrated that our son had goosebumps for the first time. His nervous system was finally processing temperature in a way it never had before.

This second round of listening therapy, including the bone conduction component (people hear through vibrations in addition to the sound waves that come through the ears), proved especially critical for Jacob's nervous system development. This more intensive treatment affected balance, visual, auditory, motor, coordination, behavior and emotional regulation skills from the first day. Jacob was not very tolerant of the vibration sensation, but we knew immediately it would be worth it. After wearing the headset for just one hour, he literally forgot how to crawl in the therapy gym floor. His motor movements became so disorganized that I had to assist the "mini-drunk man" out to the car. The progress throughout these programs was astounding, though. He started dressing and undressing himself (huge for kids who have trouble with sensory processing and poor motor planning), took an interest in learning his letters and numbers, and calmed down enough to begin learning handwriting. It was like we dug deep and hit oil — the rich benefits were going to be well worth the time and tears.

It was like we dug deep and hit oil — the rich benefits were going to be well worth the time and tears.

ASTRONAUT TRAINING

Have you ever seen a child hold their arms out, spin and spin to their heart's content, and consequently crash in the soft grass, laying there until their world finally stopped spinning? Yeah ... that wasn't Jacob. He could spin for vomit-inducing periods of time and run to the next thing that piqued his interest like it was no big deal. He had no real sense of dizziness until we started a therapy called "Astronaut Training," commonly called spin therapy. During these sessions, he sat on a large lazy-Susan-style board, and we strategically spun him to rhythmic sounds followed by eye exercises. This therapy targeted the ever important vestibular-auditory-visual triad of sensory processing. Evidently, how we experience the world heavily depends on this triad of senses working well together.

Research explains how eyes, ears and the sense of where you are in space works together as a bridge between sensory processing and motor control. This dynamic provides the backdrop for virtually *everything* we do, and its functioning affects the quality of our lives. Mrs. Hannah managed Jacob's Astronaut Training during his weekly therapy sessions, and I had a board at home with us so he could do it an additional three to five times a week as well. Through observation we discovered that Jacob's brain was reacting hypo-sensitively in the sitting up position (which is why he could typically spin for long periods of time and *not* get dizzy), but hyper-sensitively in the laying down position.

Through observation we discovered that Jacob's brain was reacting hypo-sensitively in the sitting up position (which is why he could typically spin for long periods of time and *not* get dizzy), but hyper-sensitively in the laying down position.

If Jacob hated listening therapy, he despised Astronaut Training. The first time Mrs. Hannah spun him in the laying down position and he felt disoriented to the point of looking green, he refused to get back on the board. During the second session, he dragged his feet and hands off the side of the board, interfering with the motion. After several attempts to gain his compliance, he picked up a large beach ball and threw it as hard as he could at Mrs. Hannah! It was not at all funny at the time, but now I look back and smile about how calmly she handled the attack. She said very matter-of-a-fact, "Jacob, your body and actions are telling me that you are done today. I'll see you next week."

We stuck with it though, and we started to witness a leap in mental and emotional processing. He began understanding more of what we said and started to formulate more thoughtful questions and responses. He started paying attention to his story books — seeing the pictures and hearing the stories like it was the first time, even though I had read them to him over and over again since he was born.

I have learned that there is a pyramid of functioning, and meeting sensory needs is at the bottom with logic and reasoning at the tip top. If a person doesn't get their sensory needs met in healthy ways causing them to not function well in that part of the pyramid, they can't possibly learn all the skills required to reach order, logic and reasoning.

I have learned that there is a pyramid of functioning, and meeting sensory needs is at the bottom with logic and reasoning at the tip top. If a person doesn't get their sensory needs met in healthy ways causing them to not function well in that part of the pyramid, they can't possibly learn all the skills required to reach order, logic and reasoning.

We noticed quickly that when Jacob's basic functioning improved, his emotional intelligence also leapt forward. He started caring about his relationships with people and understanding more about how his actions had a positive or negative effect on others. This newfound empathy even extended to animals. There was one day during this therapy when the kids were playing outdoors and found a baby bunny that had been killed by a neighborhood cat. Jacob was engulfed in immense grief for this tragic loss of tiny, innocent life. He wailed for nearly two hours, "BABY BUNNY! WHERE ARE YOU? BABY BUNNY! I WISH YOU WERE STILL ALIVE!" and after I had validated, and hugged, and soothed all I could … I finally did what any sensory processing disorder (SPD) mother could do. I helped him regulate with what was working for his senses at the time. I gently coaxed his blubbering self into a nice warm shower and assured him that his pain would eventually subside. After a good rhythmic pressure massage from the shower followed by a relaxing Epsom salt bath, he regulated enough to draw a sweet picture with a scrawled "B" on it in memory of the baby bunny. The next day we held a funeral under an old oak tree, and Jacob said these precious words. "Baby bunny, I wish you would come back to life. I loved you, even though I didn't know you. You were my friend."

Astronaut Training therapy led to many affectionate developments within him. He suddenly wanted to be held more and started giving us hugs and kisses. SPD kids can sometimes be so sensitive to touch that no matter how you crave love and connection as the parent, they cannot fulfill that desire. That's why I'll never forget the day he scampered out of his room after a nap, crawled into my lap and kissed my cheek. He said softly, "Mommy, I love you." The sound of those words still melts my heart to this day.

VISUAL AIDS

In addition to biomedical intervention, a sensory diet, integrative listening therapies and Astronaut Training, we also incorporated environmental aids into Jacob's daily life. This too made a positive impact on his energy levels and ability to function and communicate. Visual aids in the form of pictures (routines, meals, play options, places to go, etc.) was a major tool in our battle against sensory processing disorder (SPD).

Jacob tended to struggle with higher order thinking and executive functioning skills, which greatly impacted his quality of life. He often could not decide what to do in his free time without direction and handholding from a parent or sibling and many times had trouble following verbal directions. He also couldn't think ahead to probable consequences of any action, stop himself, and choose behavior based on the inevitable outcome. I could tell him to eat breakfast, get dressed, brush his teeth and put his shoes on until I was blue in the face, but the jobs *never* got done without me standing over him every second.

Mrs. Hannah thought it was a good idea to start using visual aids to cue his behavior, and she introduced the concept in the sensory gym to intentionally make him plan out the activities he wanted to play instead of just jumping from one thing to another like a tornado. She also provided little laminated pictures we could use on a Velcro schedule sheet at home which was labeled side-by-side with a "to do" column and a "done" column. I would line up his routine pictures for that day and as he worked the steps, he moved the matching picture to the done column. This not only calmed his anxiety about transitions, but allowed him to be able to move on to the next event with no prompting from me, which was huge for him. The visual schedule was by far the favorite tool. There were days he would carry it around like a wandering gypsy able to glimpse the future, holding it to his chest in between quick, reassuring peeks at what would come next in his day.

We also had a Velcro play time sheet that was half green and half red. I would put various toy and activity pictures for him to choose from on the green side and any off-limits activities on the red side. When he had trouble planning what to do with himself (which usually happened when I pulled away the electronic screens for a brain-break) he could visually see his green options and the no-go red ones, too. He tried to sneak his screen-time picture back on the green side occasionally, but he never got away with it!

Mrs. Hannah explained that kids with sensory processing issues don't always compute what you say. It's not that they are trying to be uninterested, distracted or are blatantly ignoring you ... they truly do not *hear and process* what you tell them to do. When you stop depending on just the auditory sense for communication and learn to communicate through multiple senses (like verbalizing that it is bath time while pointing to a visual picture of a bath), the child can "hear" you better and respond quicker with greater accuracy of the desired response. I found the visual schedule was not only a very useful tool in our home, but we also took it with us everywhere for most of his childhood including social gatherings — which had all of his SPD triggers and made his engine run high very quickly. The visual schedule gave him a sense of routine, because even when he was overwhelmed by his surroundings, he could see what was coming next, prepare for transitions and know when the chaos was going to end.

It's not that they are trying to be uninterested, distracted or are blatantly ignoring you ... they truly do not *hear* and *process* what you tell them to do.

Next to the Wilbarger Protocol, the visual schedule was a staple for us during church days. I would line up his morning routine pictures in the order of what he could expect: car, Sunday School, bathroom, church and *outside*. Requiring Jacob to sit still and quiet through church services was quite difficult for all of us, but he could see *outside* right there on his visual schedule! This strategy helped him understand what was coming and that he wouldn't have to sit still and be quiet indefinitely.

In addition to presents, the visual schedule tagged along to birthday parties as well. Some of Jacob's triggers were movement, noise and an increase in people around him. Well, what happens at parties? All three! Before we were empowered with visual aids, these triggers would lead him straight to overstimulation and meltdowns. However, when I started using the visual schedule, he could *cope*. He knew that there was a flow to the day: games, presents, cake (his slice brought from home so it was allergy-friendly) and the coveted "home" picture. Seeing what was coming broke the overwhelming event into manageable chunks for him. I also had a "sensory break" picture to fit in there any time I felt he needed heavy work or deep pressure to help keep him regulated. Before having a visual schedule, his days were a blur of anxious uncertainty and constant transition without warning. With it there was order, comfort, relaxation and a great sense of security. We could now make the environment work in our favor, which was another game changer!

Before having a visual schedule, his days were a blur of anxious uncertainty and constant transition without warning. With it there was order, comfort, relaxation and a great sense of security.

A third visual aid that helped calm our lives was a visual timer. This timer would quietly start out green, then flash yellow and beep slowly at the set warning time and would finally go red with a rapid beeping when time was up. We used this tool for those pesky transitions when he would move from a reinforcing activity to a less desirable one, like when Daddy game time was up, and bedtime was right around the corner. I would set the timer and tell him how much time he had. I would have him repeat what I had told him back to me along with what was coming up next (if he couldn't repeat it back, he wasn't processing and therefore couldn't be held responsible for further actions or reactions), and then hand him his visual schedule with the bedtime routine lined up. Jacob was not only getting verbal warnings of the transitions ahead but had a timer to remind him to get ready for the impending change, and a picture schedule to show him what was next.

With visual aids, there were no surprises to startle his nervous system. He was fully prepared. These few things simplified our lives in a very positive way. He could argue against me at times, but not against a visual timer and schedule that laid it out in black and white.

THE SPIO SUIT

Mrs. Hannah had another fabulous idea up her sleeve — the SPIO suit, which was a little lycra-vest that tightly hugged Jacob's core and provided constant deep pressure. This tool was something that could even be hidden under his clothes. It was rather expensive, but we went through an orthopedic business that could order it and fit it to Jacob, and we were able to get insurance to pick up most of the tab because we could prove (with a letter from his pediatrician and OT) that, in Jacob's case, the SPIO suit was medically necessary to stabilize his core. When he wore it in therapy sessions, he was remarkably calmer. He walked rather than careened around and was more thoughtful in general. The proprioceptive input was organizing his nervous system, thus freeing up brain space to connect in more meaningful ways to the world around him.

When Jacob was wearing his SPIO suit outside of therapy sessions, he listened better. He followed directions. He stayed in his chair at restaurants. I was so impressed I could have fallen out of my own chair! When we started letting him wear it to church, he initiated a conversation with an older member that had said "Hi" to him all his life, but he was seeing her for the first time. She was walking to her car when he ran after her saying, "Hey, you! What's your name?" He was insistent in getting her attention, and then just stood and talked to her for a moment. He suddenly had the desire to *connect* with another person instead of just running around in the grass like a wild animal released from his cage.

The SPIO suit proved beneficial in Jacob's preschool classes as well. His teachers reported that it was like night and day when he wore it. He sat more calmly in circle, seemed to listen and attend to the lessons better, and in general was more organized. Jacob wore the suit intermittently for about nine months, saving it primarily for big days involving school, church, restaurants, stores and family events. In the beginning he needed to wear it for most everything, but as time went on, he started spacing out his need for it a little at a time. Some days, he would wear it in the morning for school, take it off and get through a restaurant visit just fine, but need it back on to go to church that night. After several months, he was aware enough that the SPIO was a "crutch" of sorts, and he started to refuse it because he didn't want to be different. By this time, Jacob could identify his own needs and ask for the appropriate interventions himself, and Mrs. Hannah suggested to phase it out at his comfort level. One day I realized his SPIO had been in the bottom of his backpack for three weeks, and I had forgotten all about it. Even if insurance hadn't helped us get it, it would have been worth every penny for the calm it gave us as his nervous system continued to develop and heal.

ENVIRONMENTAL ADAPTATIONS

Some of the interventions we utilized cost money or needed an occupational therapist to direct, but environmental adaptations are completely free and easy for everyone to use. Little changes to the environment can go a long way in helping your sensational kid have a more functional, happier day.

Little changes to the environment can go a long way in helping your sensational kid have a more functional, happier day.

I remember when I first wrapped my mind around creating a sensory-friendly experience for Jacob. I kept my elderly grandmother on Fridays, and each week we would meet my parents for dinner at Cracker Barrel. Before we learned how to adapt our environment for success, we would chase Jacob around the restaurant, fighting to keep a hold of a piece of him in a sea of people, breakable displays and toys as we waited to be seated. Many times, Eric or I had to scoop up a distraught child and carry him to the table when our name was called. I could feel the stares boring into my back, and my temper would start to rise. One evening he struggled loose in my arms when we were walking in between two tables, and he ended up shattering one of their lamp globes. I could feel the judgement from others as they spoke through their eyes, "Look at that kid misbehave! She really needs to discipline and show him who is boss." Don't we *honestly* all think that when we see an unruly kid in public? I fought these contradicting emotions — part of me wanted to discipline to make *me* feel better, and the other part of me knew it wouldn't help a lick. Once we got to the table, we would pin him in between two adults and take turns sitting him down, dragging his hands away from things and covering his loud mouth ... oh, and we ate dinner in between! As if that wasn't exhausting enough, the car ride home claimed the last bit of our sanity as Jacob, vibrating with energy, melted down into a screaming, crying puddle of exhaustion.

Through therapy and research, I got sensory-smart, and we changed the game plan yet again. Our first successful Friday night dinner experience came when I took a toy drum that lit up and played music in the car with us. This toy gave him some proprioceptive, auditory and visual stimulation on the way to the restaurant. I purposefully filled up his "sensory bucket" so he could be more regulated once we got to our destination. While we were waiting, we let him open the heavy door for people going in and out. This give him heavy work, and a good dose of self-confidence with numerous smiles and gracious compliments. I could see his little chest swell with pride at these positive responses, especially since he was so accustomed to correction. When he tired of that, Eric and I let him walk up our legs and flip over backwards repeatedly for vestibular input, and then we told him to pretend he was glued to the nearby pole and hold on tight. He laughed and held on with all his might as we pulled on him. Sure, people stared, but who cared? When our name was called, the rest of my family went to the table first and got settled, which prevented Jacob and me having to slowly move through the mess of people and tempting displays like Friday night cattle. Then I walked him in and allowed him to choose one display to look at before sitting down, and I promised him that we could take a peek at the toy section after dinner. I brought a gamut of wind-up toys and Play-Doh for fine motor work at the table, and we all got to *eat* in relative peace. My mother then took him to the toys while Eric and I paid the bill, and then out to the car we went. I was giddy with excitement of a plan well-executed.

Through therapy and research, I got sensory-smart, and we changed the game plan yet again.

Environmental adaptations became like the sensory diet for us. We had to figure out what Jacob needed at that season of life and accommodate the best we could. Our main focus as he grew was to teach him to ask for what he needed and save us the guess work. Some other adaptations for Jacob included a weighted blanket (which we used for bedtime and church), adjusting lighting when necessary and acquiring a pair of noise-cancellation headphones for loud places. We also allowed him to watch a favorite video or listen to music from our phones with earbuds in, especially at cousins' musical concerts or school programs. While a lot of people frown on screen time, I believe in moderation and at the right times it actually gives his brain a *break* from processing all the noise and movement going on. When he unplugged again, he was more organized and ready to reengage in his environment. So, for us, it was a win-win.

It also was not beyond us to ask for the volume to be turned down in restaurants or tell him to cover his nose with his shirt and "smell home" as we hurried by the perfume counter at the mall. The stickiest challenge was how to modify foods he found aversive in order to not hurt people's feelings. When others offered him food or asked why he wasn't eating, we taught him to reply with catch phrases like, "I appreciate it, but no thank you," and even "I appreciate your opinion, but I respectfully disagree." The last phrase was tongue-in-cheek for those people (we all know them) who just don't give up with the food stuff! I mean, why is it such a big deal to *you* if my child isn't eating? Obviously, he isn't starved.

Let me explain something about sensory kids being picky eaters. It's not always their choice to be obstinate and so very frustrating. Picky eating has little to do with taste (since we can only taste five flavors anyway) and everything to do with smell and texture. Smell is one of our oldest primal senses, designed to keep us safe. Think of how you would grab your nose and run from noxious odors like putrid spoiled meat. You would innately know that if you ingested something that smelled so awful, it would make you very ill and possibly even kill you! I don't imagine, even when forced, you could get a piece of rotten meat to your tongue before gagging and losing stomach contents. Sensory kids also have this very strong flight response, but here's the kicker — it's in response to *normal* food. Their brain is misinterpreting the sensory signals from their body again. What we see as normal, they see as noxiously life-threatening. No wonder food wars ensue. The times we tried to force food in Jacob ended with vomit and apologies. Once I learned to adapt our environment to our needs, however, I carried a lunch box of Jacob-approved food everywhere. If he couldn't eat what was served, he ate from his lunch box. If he couldn't even stomach his lunch box food because other stimuli were too invasive at the moment, he just didn't eat until he was back in the comforts of the car or home. I promise you your kid will not starve. They will eat when their sensory systems settle down and food becomes appealing again.

Let me explain something about sensory kids being picky eaters. It's not always their choice to be obstinate and so very frustrating.

JACOB'S DREAM LUNCHBOX

Every person's food allergies, sensitivities and preferences vary, but here is a glimpse of how personal food management can be done. Whether we are headed to a party away from home, we are hosting a holiday or event in-home or going out-of-town, if food will be served, we pack Jacob's lunchbox.

For holidays and events away from home:

We pack the following and find a quiet place to snack when hungry: gluten-free protein bar of choice at the time, apple-sauce, raisins, dye-free fruit snacks, chips of choice (they even make dye-free Doritos!), dye-free wintergreen mints, dye-free juice pouches, and a treat (dye-free sucker or licorice, or gluten-free cookies).

For birthday parties where there will be dessert he cannot have, I make sure he has gluten-free cake and fruit sorbet (we have a mini-freezer pack that works well for these frozen add-ins).

When we host parties in the home:

All of the above is packed in his lunchbox and placed in his bedroom, where he is allowed to eat by himself when he is hungry. This allows him to avoid crowds and smells. It's also a plus because we have access to our oven and fridge, which means when the party dies down, I can throw his favorite gluten-free chicken nuggets in the oven and he gets a dye-free popsicle for dessert.

Trips and Vacations:

We make his favorite foods (like gluten-free pancakes) in bulk and pack those along with bought beverages (like almond-based chocolate milk) and boxes of snacks in coolers and bags. If the destination is close, we drive straight through and change ice in the coolers as needed. If we stay overnight, we make sure the hotel has a mini fridge. If we are going to be gone for a week or longer, we do all of the above AND a grocery run (pre-order click-lists are great) and stay in a condo with oven and fridge access.

For some reason, adapting the environment for the tactile sense was the most difficult to wrap my mind and heart around. Sensory kids can be very conscientious about what touches their body. The notorious naysayers who refuse to even recognize sensory processing disorder (SPD) as a legitimate disorder complain that we are just letting the tail wag the dog on this one (along with every other modification). But in truth, normal fabrics and textures can actually produce a pain signal in the brain for these kids.

For some reason, adapting the environment for the tactile sense was the most difficult to wrap my mind and heart around.

When I understood this struggle with Jacob — that he wasn't just being fussy and difficult — we stopped pushing the offending clothes like button-up shirts, cute holiday three-piece suits, khaki pants and even most types of footwear. They made him utterly *miserable* (assuming we were even able to wrestle those clothes on him that given day), and in return he made the family's day miserable with continual whining, complaining, pulling and tugging. Now that I have knowledge that allows me to empathize, I choose to invest in softer alternatives with elastic waistbands and fewer seams. We also allow him to occasionally sleep in the clothes he will wear the next day, especially if we will be getting up early the next morning. This "breaks in" his clothes and makes them very comfortable on his skin. It also helps avoid the hectic morning rush to get him up and dressed into new, crisp clothes that may be assaulting to his waking nervous system. Who cares if they have a few extra wrinkles? Not us! What was hard about letting go of the clothes war was letting go of the *expectations* attached to it.

You see, since Jacob was a baby, I tried to put him in blue jeans. I mean, doesn't everyone wear blue jeans? They're cute ... they're American ... and they exude *typical*. When I realized blue jeans, with all those little seams and stiffness around the pockets and waist, were actually *hurting* him, I tucked them in the back of his drawer. I secretly hoped that we would beat this neurological wrinkle in our lives, and then the blue jeans could come back to the front of the drawer where they belonged, and all would be right with the world.

Months went by, and I decided to buy the softest, secondhand pairs of jeans possible. I mean, these jeans had been washed until nearly threadbare. But Jacob couldn't tolerate those either. I put all of the jeans in storage bags and left them in the basement for a year or two. We just needed more time. We needed more occupational therapy and biomedical intervention. We needed to fix how his brain worked. We needed to fix *him*. The blue jeans would then be able to resurface. I remember the weekend I cleaned out the laundry room and found countless pairs of little blue jeans, all different sizes. I sat on the cold concrete basement floor and held them in my hands. I smelled them. I felt them on my face. I debated putting them back in the bag or giving them to charity. Should I hold on or let go? My heart ached when I allowed myself to honestly admit he would probably *never* wear them. He would never be like everyone else ... then it hit me. I didn't *want* him to be like everyone else. I still don't want any other kid. This one is beyond ordinary, and he is mine.

He would never be like everyone else ... then it hit me. I didn't *want* him to be like everyone else. I still don't want any other kid. This one is beyond ordinary, and he is mine.

The art of environmental adaptations taught me that I didn't need a boy who was happy in blue jeans. I just needed the boy ... happy to be alive, happy to love and help others, happy to learn from the world. I wanted a young man who would discover what really matters in life. I yearned for an adult son who never forgets the privilege and mercy that God bestows upon him. I needed a well-rounded person who values his strengths and works within them, knowing how to minimize his weaknesses without minimizing his self-esteem. I just wanted a boy who was happy in general because he knows he is *perfect* just the way God made him.

Occupational therapists are a great help when it comes to thinking of ways to adapt your environment, like we did ours. Use their expertise and your own detective work and grow confident in a new reality for your sensational loved ones today. And remember, these kinds of changes are completely free!

A QUICK WORD TO GAMERS

You read that environmental adaptations are like part of the sensory diet — you have to figure out what to put in at what time to help your loved one be more functional. However, the other side of that coin is also learning when to take whichever stimulation *out* of the diet.

Screens, screens, and more screens... oh, my!

It is a fact that we live in a technology-saturated environment, and that is not going to change. There are many studies about how technology affects the brain and nervous system, and even though there are a few pros, I found it interesting to learn the science behind what we already know in our gut — screen time most definitely has a *negative* impact on SPD. If you want to read up on the topic, check out the book *Glow Kids: How Screen Addiction is Hijacking Our Kids – and How to Break the Trance* by Nicholas Kardaras. Screen time takes you out of reality and experiencing life through your *whole* body and substitutes your experiential knowledge through just your visual and auditory senses. This means your proprioceptive, vestibular and tactile senses get very little workout, which results in — you got it — a *dulled* sensory system. This is never good considering people with SPD already have impaired nervous systems to start with! So, do I let Jacob play screens? *Yes* ... of course. I just work extra hard to monitor and modify his usage. The pediatrician recommends two hours of screen time daily. We do good to cut it to four hours, realistically. But when Jacob starts having more irritable days and night-waking, we know we've indulged too much, and it's time to give his body a technology detox.

How do we fight the screen battle?

- We have very honest conversations about what screen time does to our brain. Jacob knows how it contributes to his attention deficit and hyperactivity disorder (ADHD) symptoms *and* overstimulates his nervous system.

- We alternate screen time with *brain breaks*, where you have to do other things with your mind and body (preferably outside where all the senses can be exercised).

- We set rules on how much screen time we have in a day, and within that, how much of the allotted time goes to whichever screen (online gaming, video-streaming, or in-home gaming systems).

- All family members practice times of "screens down" (even adults with their phones) usually at meals, restaurants, car rides and when we need to be tuned into family and friends.

- Screens go off after dinner to allow for movement activities and reading books before settling into bed.

BRAIN TRAINING

Another intervention that worked miracles for us, outside of occupational therapy, was a local brain training program. This franchise claimed they could improve cognitive function through specific brain training techniques, and for Jacob, they most certainly did. Jacob had so many executive functioning issues that were inhibiting his higher order thinking, especially by the time he was school-aged and had academic work to do. During this program, I saw huge gains in his visual memory, auditory processing, logic and reasoning skills, processing speed, attention and handwriting.

Before brain training, I worried much about Jacob's learning ability. Would he ever be able to segment sounds to spell? Think about the steps required. Cat is c-a-t, which you must be able to hear each sound, know which letter makes that sound, and hold it all in your mind long enough to write it out. As kindergarten got closer, I laid awake at night, wondering what we would do if he couldn't learn to read *or* write. He had auditory issues and significant fine motor delays that kept his hand from holding and controlling a pencil for any length of time. After brain training, my worries just melted away. Sensory processing disorder (SPD) finally took a backseat, and our lives got on track once and for all from the train wreck that almost derailed our family.

**After brain training, my worries just melted away.
Sensory processing disorder (SPD) finally took
a backseat, and our lives got on track once and for all
from the train wreck that almost derailed our family.**

Like interactive listening therapies, brain training was grueling day-to-day work. There were home components, and long after the sessions ended, I continued the home program. When he started reading, writing and spelling, I breathed a huge sigh of relief. Another intervention well worth our time, effort and money. Now he has a book in his hand nearly all day, and while he may never have *neat* handwriting (do boys generally have neat handwriting?), his thoughts are well constructed and legible. The benefits just kept piling up long after all these programs were completed!

INTERACTIVE METRONOME TRAINING

Interactive Metronome (IM) training is a computer-based program that he used through his occupational therapy center that focused on improving timing, attention and coordination. Out of all the therapies and trainings he did, this one was actually pleasing to Jacob. It literally had him clapping and moving his feet in rhythm in simple to complex methods, and while it exhausted him mentally and physically, he enjoyed this type of work.

Rhythm is amazing for the body and brain. It synchronizes brain waves and with it comes a greater level of sensory integration and body awareness. There is nothing like mind and body being in sync. By learning to keep beat, the brain learns to plan, sequence and process more efficiently.

Rhythm is amazing for the body and brain. It synchronizes brain waves and with it comes a greater level of sensory integration and body awareness.

IM training had its challenging moments, but it was icing on the cake for us. By the time he finished the sessions, we had seen marked improvement in Jacob's attention and focus, motor control/

coordination, language processing, reading and math fluency, and his continued ability to regulate impulsivity. If the integrative listening programs hadn't sold me on the beautiful relationship between music and the brain, this sure did! Jacob actually picked up some drum lessons after that. I still smile every time I hear him tap out various rhythms, and I beamed with pride when he performed at a talent show on the drums. He doesn't fully realize he is continuing this important brain work, and I'm not going to let that secret slip.

THE CRAWLING PROGRAM

We were beginning to see the light at the end of the tunnel when my best friend asked me to read a book about a crawling program she had stumbled upon. *Stopping ADHD: A Unique and Proven Drug-Free Program for Treating ADHD in Children and Adults* by Nancy E. O'Dell, PhD. and Patricia A. Cook, PhD. did not disappoint. I read and studied it, and then showed it to Mrs. Hannah, who said it wouldn't hurt to give their ideas a try. The book talked mostly about the Symmetric Tonic Neck Reflex (STNR) and how if children hadn't learned how to crawl properly as a baby, they may have a few unresolved reflexes that could still be affecting their development.

Jacob had crawled on one knee, the other knee up as he pushed along with his foot. He crawled for a very short time period before he just started walking (and bumping and crashing). I remembered vividly how, at church, if we tried to cross his legs or push them down from waving in the air, his arms would fling out and hit my mom and me in the stomachs. Likewise, if we tried to control his arms, his legs would go wild, thumping the bench full of people in front of us! Resolving this STNR Reflex (and other unresolved reflexes from infancy) through various crawling exercises could better integrate the motor and sensory systems. Who knew crawling was *so* important?

Resolving this STNR Reflex (and other unresolved reflexes from infancy) through various crawling exercises could better integrate the motor and sensory systems. Who knew crawling was so important?

Like some of the other intense interventions, this one also took a whole lot of time and dedication. There were days neither of us wanted to go downstairs and do the crawling exercises, but we mustered resolve and did it anyway. It *was* fascinating to watch Jacob struggle across the floor on all fours, though, trying to move the right side of his body and then the left, almost in a stiff and robotic in motion. He even had trouble holding his head up so he could see where he was going! Wouldn't you say there were some unresolved issues there? He slowly got the hang of alternating his hands with his opposite knees, and eventually he did retrain his body to crawl around as fast and fluidly as any 10-month-old I'd ever seen (at the age of 6!).

About that time, we had exceeded our set goals in OT as well. Mrs. Hannah was ready to release us. It was a bittersweet farewell, but she said we could always contact her with any questions, assuring me she would always be there for us. And she has been — even for the writing of this book! I didn't have to reach back out for much OT help, however. When doctors, OTs and family had done their jobs well, we were ready to soar and not look back.

ADHD MEDICATIONS

You should know that I completely exhausted every avenue of treatment before turning to prescribed medicine. I wanted to feel confident that I had explored all our options first. Then, if medication was necessary, we could add it in only if we *had* to. There came a time, after all interventions were finished and we had been homeschooling multiple years, that Jacob's attention deficits and hyperactivity were impeding additional progress. He still felt disorganized in his own mind and body, so we decided to give medications a try. It was like night and day for us all!

He still felt disorganized in his own mind and body, so we decided to give medications a try. It was like night and day for us all!

We worked with the pediatrician to find the appropriate medication and dosage amount, taking advantage of the cheek swab test that told us which medications could work in his body, and suddenly Jacob had more self-control and could get his work done in a third of the time. If I forgot to include the pill with his morning vitamins on school days, he would realize he was struggling in a subject and ask for it. He had grown to be so introspective that he knew when it wasn't in his system because he could identify what scattered and not scattered felt like now.

Most importantly, the attention deficit and hyperactivity disorder (ADHD) medication helped organize him enough that he could continue learning skills and concepts needed for adolescence and beyond. If you have tried multiple interventions and think ADHD medications could help your child, research the benefits and risks for yourself, and be sure to talk to your doctor. Jacob will probably need a little something extra off and on throughout his life, but at this point, it's been the golden ticket in helping him attend and meet age-appropriate academic and social expectations.

MARTIAL ARTS

When Jacob was at his best, thriving in the home and school fronts, Taekwondo was the last "therapy" we incorporated. Martial arts of all kinds are proven to increase body awareness, control, attention and focus — all of which are diminished in children with nervous system conditions like attention deficit (hyperactivity) disorder (ADD/ADHD), autism and sensory processing disorder (SPD).

Jacob showed an interest and focus with martial arts that I had never seen before. From the first class he was engaged, listening and giving his best effort, which was amazing given it took place in an extraordinarily loud room with a ton of movement going on around him! He didn't get distracted that the group next to him was doing a different form or technique, nor did the yelling, smacking of equipment, or ringing gongs damper his fun. He was "in the zone" and I was in happy tears on the sidelines.

I watched his patient instructors work with him on body awareness and control within the skilled movement techniques, and the benefits carried over into home life. I watched his classmates encourage him, and I saw his confidence and self-esteem grow in all areas. The best part was when the director personally invited him to participate in their annual Hwangs Martial Arts World Taekwondo Championship Tournament, telling him (and me) she was *sure* he could do it. This involved him being in a massive crowd of people, sitting on the stadium floor, listening and engaged for three long hours, while his sensory-supportive entourage sat in the seating sections far out of reach. I didn't want to let him do it at first, but when he looked at me with pleading eyes, I knew this was a make it or break it moment. Either I believed in him, or I didn't. So, I packed him a sensory backpack, and together our family made the leap into something new and unpredictable.

I still remember the marvelous feeling, sitting on the sidelines, watching my child succeed without me. That had been the goal all along, and we finally achieved it. Not only did he not need the backpack, but he succeeded with only one minor meltdown set off while transitioning from the bleachers to the packed stadium floor in a sea of people. He panicked when he realized he didn't know exactly where to go and ran back to me in tears, saying he wanted to go home. Thankfully, a volunteer who had raised a son with autism herself saw me trying to calm and direct him, tears streaming down his face, and she wrapped her arm around him and with a gentle squeeze said she'd take him right to his group for the opening parade and all would be well. His anxiety calmed immediately and it was my turn to tear up. Jacob gave that tournament his all and brought home a second-place medal, trophy and a smile that was priceless!

I still remember the marvelous feeling, sitting on the sidelines, watching my child succeed without me. That had been the goal all along, and we finally achieved it.

Without the biomedical intervention, diet changes and various therapies to initially heal Jacob's nervous system, I do not think martial arts would have helped further Jacob's overall success. The noise would have hurt his ears. The crowds and movement would have triggered debilitating overstimulation. His body wouldn't have been able to get in or hold the proper positions because of lack of motor control and coordination. But because SPD is now farther behind us, I know he can go out and do any activity he chooses — do anything he wants in his life — and that is worth all the hard work and effort, hands down!

THE SKINNY ON COST AND TIME COMMITMENTS

We implemented 14 different interventions with Jacob from the time of his diagnosis — working intensely for over three years and then intermittently (continuing lifestyle changes mostly) after that. So how far in the ground did that run us financially? When I say we worked *intensely*, what kind of time commitment am I talking about? Are interventions like these even feasible for you, or are you considering closing this book and giving up? My first hope is that you don't stop now. Instead, my answer is keep exploring what is possible for *you*, and definitely read on!

COST EXPECTATIONS & TIME COMMITMENTS

The most expensive intervention for us, hands down, was biomedical intervention. We found that most holistic integrationists did not take insurance and the expense was out of pocket. Luckily, my husband had amazing insurance that picked up most of the blood work cost even though it did not pick up the $300 office visits. With three office visits plus the urine, stool, blood and genetic testing we did initially, our first year of biomedical intervention cost us approximately $4,000 which included implementing the customized vitamin regimen that he began monthly. We didn't do as much testing for subsequent years, however, and once he was well on track, we only had one office visit for a yearly check-up. At that point, we spent approximately $2,500 a year which included the continued vitamin regimen. While this intervention is expensive, it takes minimal time — besides a doctor appointment, hospital trip for tests and packing pills — and now all I have to do is remember to give him the vitamins!

Accommodating the food allergies, which is really an extension of biomedical intervention, is also rather expensive. Initially, it took time and money for us to switch out the food in our house and wrap our minds around what allergy-friendly foods we could substitute with (it was a trial and error for a while to see what Jacob would eat). Then we turned our attention to allergy-free household products, and it is no secret that buying organic and natural products drains the pocketbook. This accommodation probably doubled, if not tripled, our grocery bill. Once we took the plunge, it became a lifestyle change and the time commitment is only packing a lunchbox as needed.

Brain Training was the next most expensive venture. This particular program cost us approximately $1,300. We invested in a session a week for about six months and did follow up exercises at home. Overall, our time commitment was about four to five hours a week for half a year. The great part was that they let us keep the exercise materials for in-home review, which we take advantage of from time to time to keep the targeted skills sharpened.

Occupational therapy has the potential to be pricey depending upon your insurance. Our insurance allowed us a certain number of visits each year, which allowed us to go one to two times per week at no out-of-pocket cost. Mrs. Hannah and the administration knew how many visits we were allowed, so we divided them through the year and never ran out of our allotted sessions.

Several of our interventions were done through occupational therapy, but the SPIO suit did require additional cost. Without insurance, we would have been expected to pay between $150 - $300, but with our insurance, we were able to purchase the suit for $80.

Interactive listening programs run around $1,500, but our therapy center had bought systems to rent to their clients for about $100 a month, saving us in the long run. Likewise, we used the Interactive Metronome (IM) training through the therapy center as well and because they administered the sessions on site, we paid nothing for this intervention. If you tried to buy the IM equipment and program to utilize in-home on your own, it could cost $1,000 - $2,000 easily!

The Wilbarger Protocol required the cost of a brush (which is minimal), and the sensory diet, visual aids and environmental adaptations also had a one-time-cost to get initial materials up and running in the home, but none of it was very expensive and a lot was completely free. Astronaut Training could have been the cost of a large Lazy-Susan style board, but we borrowed one from the therapy center for the length of the program which saved us money. The crawling program, which I implemented on my own from a book (under his therapist's approval), was also free.

Medicine for attention deficit and hyperactivity disorder (ADHD) varies in price depending upon which medication you utilize and your insurance coverage. The first one we tried was $75 per month. Thankfully that one made him nauseous, which prompted us to try a different option for only $10 a month (a price-point we could better manage). We did do a check-swab test initially to tell us by his genetics which couple of medications would work best in his body, and that was a one-time $100 out of pocket expense. Insurance typically does not cover the expense of that test, but because of

Jacob's slow detox system, we were unwilling to put a drug in his body that may have adverse effects for an unnaturally long period of time. We did apply to insurance to have them cover the swab test, and in our case, they did pick up the cost.

While therapy did not turn out to be too expensive for my family, it was certainly time consuming. Each program we tried typically took a few months each to execute — some programs overlapping and some running back-to-back. It seemed like my life spun in place for those three-and-a-half years as we got Jacob the help he needed. I did not move forward ... I did not pass go. I ate, slept and breathed OT. From the time we woke up to the time we went to bed, we were implementing whichever program at the therapy center and following up at home. It became part of our lifestyle to handle every behavior and situation as a therapist would. Time consuming doesn't even cover it ... for us it was *life-changing*, never again to be the same.

Time consuming doesn't even cover it ... for us it was *life-changing*, never again to be the same.

Now, of course I believe that all these interventions were worth *our* money and time, but that doesn't mean it will be for you. I am a stay-at-home mother with the time to devote, and my husband has a job with a salary and insurance coverage that could support our efforts. There were some tight financial months early on, where we had to watch our spending habits and cut out luxuries, but for the most part we came through this whole experience financially intact. Your situation and experience could be completely different, and that's okay!

Whether you can afford the time and energy to do all of these options and more (yes, there is *more* we couldn't or didn't do), or you wonder if you have the capacity to make a difference — there is still hope, and there are things you *can* do to help your child.

Whether you can afford the time and energy to do all of these options and more (yes, there is *more* we couldn't or didn't do), or you wonder if you have the capacity to make a difference — there is still hope, and there are things you *can* do to help your child.

WHERE TO START

I believe that it is *most* important to first and foremost find an occupational therapist, even if you pay for sessions out of pocket for a short period of time. OTs have the knowledge and tools to get you started at home with sensory diets, visual aids and environmental adaptations — the mostly free options that will be the most bang for your buck. Once you learn about sensory processing disorder (SPD) and how to better help your child (and teach them to help themselves), you'll always have the knowledge and tools to continue at home when money runs out. Every step forward is moving your family in the right direction. If your budget allows, you can continue utilizing OT, always learning new things to add to your toolbox.

If you can have the option to try a biomedical intervention, I suggest that you start by changing your child's diet first as it will make the largest impact on the interdependent gastrointestinal-immune-nervous systems. Take it slow and consider changing out one food at a time ... then one product at a time. Start by omitting gluten and dairy. Then if budget allows, keep cleaning up the diet and look for an integrationist who check for harmful bacteria, metal exposure and levels of key vitamins, minerals and antioxidants that affect overall nervous system function.

The bottom line is do what *you* can do with the time and resources *you* have. Just don't give up. Every little change will add up to a positive impact for the body and brain!

INTERVENTIONS BY AGE AND COST

No matter how old you or your loved one is, there are lifestyle changes you can make to improve functioning and quality of life. See my OT-approved list of suggestions below for ideas.

Key

*	Cost of materials	No $ sign	Free
**	OT guidance is recommended to get started or for duration	$	Inexpensive
		$$	Minimally Expensive
		$$$	Expensive
***	Doctor supervision		

Young Child	Older Child/ Teenager	Adult
Environmental Adaptations	Environmental Adaptations	Environmental Adaptations
Sensory Diet **	Sensory Diet **	Sensory Diet **
The Crawling Program $*	The Crawling Program $*	The Crawling Program $*
Visual Aids $*	Visual Aids $*	Visual Aids $*
Wilbarger Protocol $**	Wilbarger Protocol $**	Wilbarger Protocol $*
Integrative Listening Therapy $$**	Integrative Listening Therapy $$**	Integrative Listening Therapy $$**
Astronaut Training $**	Astronaut Training $**	---
ADHD Medications $$***	ADHD Medications $$***	ADHD Medications $$***
SPIO Suit $$*	SPIO Suit $$*	SPIO Suit $$*
Brain Training Programs $$	Brain Training Programs $$	Brain Training Programs $$
Interactive Metronome Training $$**	Interactive Metronome Training $$**	Interactive Metronome Training $$*
Allergy-Free Diet $$	Allergy-Free Diet $$	Allergy-Free Diet $$
Biomedical Intervention $$$***	Biomedical Intervention $$$***	Biomedical Intervention $$$***
Martial Arts $$$	Martial Arts $$$	Martial Arts $$$

Hannah's Professional Opinion

Do you think healthy, allergy-free nutrition helps sensory processing disorder (SPD)?

I am a huge proponent of healthy nutrition, partly because I was lucky enough to be raised by a family who taught me that what you feed yourself is important. It is difficult in our culture — with its relationship to food — to eat healthy, especially with all the sugar and junk food that is pushed at us. There is a lot of research that supports how what you eat most definitely affects gut, brain and immune health.

Overall, I believe a healthy diet helps my clients. However, since my focus is occupational therapy, it is difficult to say how much diet influences a child's behavior, attention and state of arousal or awareness of surroundings, because nutrition is only one part of a multi-faceted treatment program. Some kids I know, like Jacob, have definite allergies to food that when ingested negatively affect his behavior and attention. It's really important for families to research, learn and understand their child's body and what impacts it negatively, if anything.

If a family wants to pursue this important piece of treatment for their child, I recommend they literally go with their gut.

Why are sensory diets such an integral part of occupational therapy (OT) intervention?

If you have kids with SPD, attention deficit (hyperactivity) disorder (ADD/ADHD) or autism, a sensory diet has to do with movement and sensory experiences that help them feel better so they can function optimally. The strategies taught can help them learn to self-regulate as children and grow into coping skills for adulthood. We all have needs that have to be met for us to feel good and function at our best, so a sensory diet is actively creating an awareness of what it is that you need and how to provide for those needs in the best way at the best time. It's a type of investigative process that we can use all our lives to keep ourselves mentally, emotionally and physically healthy.

Why might OTs be more qualified to set up a sensory diet than a parent?

Parents can research and educate themselves on their own, but therapists have been to school and continue to go to seminars to understand these disorders and how to treat them to improve quality of life. There is new research and cutting-edge interventions coming out all the time, and part of being a therapist is knowing the best treatment plan to offer. Plus, every individual child is different and may need different plans. What works for one child may not work for another. What works today may not work tomorrow. Parents do not need to take on the world by themselves. Utilize the professionals who can make life easier when possible.

What can happen if a parent tries to accommodate needs without a therapist's expertise?

Parents may learn just enough to be dangerous. For instance, they may identify their child needs to spin to satisfy their vestibular need. If you do not know how long to spin them or in what direction (circular or linear, for example), you can unintentionally overstimulate the child which is not the desired outcome. Therapists can teach parents what hypersensitivity or overstimulation looks like (some signs are so subtle and easy to misinterpret) and how to give which kind of input at appropriate levels to get the optimal result for the child. If you are not highly educated in the field, you can accidently be counterproductive and ruin the sensory diet experience for the child. If the kid gets sick every time they spin because they are becoming overstimulated, they may never want to spin again when spinning could have been a valuable tool for self-regulation, if done correctly to start with.

Are integrative listening therapies and Astronaut Training easy to incorporate into OT programs?

The concept of Astronaut Training is amazing, because it works on the visual-auditory-vestibular triad that is so important for how you move through space. For there to be a program that works to incorporate all three of those together is fascinating, but I've found it is difficult for parents to find the time to carry through at home for a long enough period of time for it to yield results. That's another reason why it is a good idea to work with a therapist for some of these programs.

Now, based on my experience, integrated listening therapies are easier for parents and yield quicker results, and there are several listening programs available. It is more auditory-based, and there is just something to music — and modulated music — that really helps brain function. You can also incorporate exercises to target the visual system and movement to target the vestibular system, to work on the triad that has been mentioned.

What was your view of watching Jacob go through these changes?

Jacob often bulldozed into the room. He was loud, aggressive, inattentive and wasn't at all aware of his body or what anyone else's body was doing. During the first round of listening therapy he was so high energy, and because of his explosiveness and need for movement, it was hard for him to slow down and "be present," meaning he was so driven by his body's need for stimuli that he barely noticed others in the room let alone have the ability to interact with them. I remember when he started to self-actualize and be more present in the moment. He became calm and attentive, and then he could interact more purposefully with less destruction which meant he could start forming relationships with the people around him.

Should parents always adapt the environment to fit their child's needs?

All the strategies mentioned help a child when behaviors get really intense. When you communicate and show them plans or transitions that are coming up, it helps them feel safer. Visual schedules, especially, give them some control and serve to eliminate undue stress. These kids generally need to know what is going on so they can prepare their bodies for it. I highly recommend a lot of preparation in the beginning of intervention. Then, as you progress through treatment, it is a good idea to throw in unexpected pieces now and again because that is how kids will slowly start to learn to manage their own sensory needs and when to regulate themselves. Unexpected changes to schedules are difficult and traumatic, and it can increase anxiety, frustration and negative behaviors, but as they grow and learn how to adapt it is important that they practice appropriate responses. Then they can self-calm in the future.

Why are Interactive Metronome (IM) trainings so helpful with SPD?

IM training improves nervous system functioning in the forms of cognitive and motor skills across the board. Even adults with traumatic brain injuries can benefit from IM. Within the framework of SPD, and in Jacob's case, I used IM in hopes to address attention, motor planning coordination and organization of his overall nervous system where the brain-body connection was concerned. There is research that demonstrates IM enhances somatosensory discrimination to increase body scheme awareness. I think, whether through proprioception or the motor movement repetition (which targets bilateral coordination, timing and sequencing), IM did help increase Jacob's attention span and improve his motor planning coordination. Most importantly, we saw how much more organized and calm he seemed after his sessions.

How can learning to crawl really matter?

Crawling develops bilateral coordination which activates both sides of the brain, and the weight bearing/proprioceptive input (especially on the upper body) develops proximal stability. Proximal stability refers to your core trunk and shoulder control, which is the building block for future distal mobility (fine motor skills, like handwriting). Crawling also strengthens all the muscles to meet the needs of toddlerhood, while integrating the last of the reflexes left from birth.

Those primitive reflexes initially help you develop coordinated motor movements or patterns, which is important for an infant, but if they persist into later life, they can cause a lot of motor problems. Motor complications can end up negatively affecting the sensory system which may further impact behavior. As your proximal stability increases, you no longer demonstrate the influence of primitive reflexive movement patterns which allows you to gain more control over your body and develop more mature motor patterns. That being said, many people do lead functional lives even if they don't crawl. In my opinion, if a child learns to crawl they will increase the connections between both sides of the brain, which assists with overall coordination and well-rounded brain function.

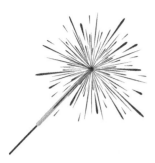

PART THREE

ATTITUDES THAT MADE THE DIFFERENCE

Forget the Naysayers

Hannah's Professional Opinion

PLAN FOR SUCCESS

Nothing is more fun for our family than holidays and vacations. Done up well, even sensory kids can enjoy these out of routine experiences.

The catch phrase to memorize is "*adjust* the expectations and *plan* for success." The truth is, if you are observant and respectful of your child's needs and plan accordingly, the whole family *can* have fun. Preventing sensory meltdowns has always been our focus, but planning for success also means giving thought to how we respond if the train does go off the track.

The catch phrase to memorize is "*adjust* the expectations and *plan* for success."

I call it "what if planning," and I realize it can be overwhelming. When we travel, meals are the first thing I mentally and physically prep for. I always ensure we have "Jacob's Dream Lunchbox" ready because if Jacob is accidentally poisoned by allergens, it ruins the vacation for everyone! Planning for success means researching the area we will frequent for restaurants he can eat at and then planning our pit stops and hotel stays accordingly. I also pack as much food as possible from home and make sure the hotels have mini-fridges and microwaves, or we opt to stay in condos with a full kitchen.

Remember also that when out of routine, sensory kids cannot always eat what is offered, or eat *when* it is offered. For instance, we went to Disney World when Jacob was 6. For a whole week he basically ate gluten-free Mickey Mouse waffles and French fries for *every* meal! Many vacation days end with Jacob grazing in the hotel room at bedtime, because he barely ate meals with the rest of us during the day. We had learned quickly to adjust our expectations to accommodate this probability, and packed extra healthy snacks for when the sensory overload subsided, and he settled enough to feel hungry.

Vacations are full of sensory processing disorder (SPD) triggers, and feeding issues are just one of the many you must think about ahead of time. There are changes in routine and new experiences. There are transitions and the need for being flexible with plans. There are also sensory sensitivities, modulation issues and impulsivity spikes. One of the greatest vacations I ever pulled off was a trip to the beach with my best friend's family. We had two sensory-smart mommas, two patient husbands, and three kids – *two* of those with SPD (mine is a sensory-seeker while hers is a sensory-avoider). How in the world did we do it? We adjusted our expectations and fully understood the undertaking, and then we planned out the wazoo.

We knew our children well. She told her daughter about the trip months in advance and showed her the condo pictures and pictures of all the places we would probably go for meals and fun time. As an avoider, her daughter needed to be fully equipped and prepared. She needed to walk through the trip and all the possibilities a million times in her mind. In contrast, I didn't tell my sensory seeker we were going until one month before and then hung a visual countdown poster on the wall so the kids could put a stamp on each day from 30 down to one. Jacob would have driven me *crazy*, and his energy would have been through the roof if he knew too early and had to wait too long. Our families also decided to drive 12 hours straight through to Alabama to avoid hotel transitions. We packed sensory toys like bubbles, a bat, ball and frisbee and planned multiple rest area stops to allow for movement and sensory regulation throughout the very long traveling day. They were headed toward a meltdown during one driving stretch, so we adjusted expectations, pulled over in a store parking lot, and let them play a rousing game of "don't touch the ground" as they climbed all over the bars of a large cart return caddy! When we arrived at the condo, we immediately set up sensory hideouts in most rooms, being mindful of the extroverts who needed hands-on activities and the introverts who needed quiet time and soft book nooks. Our hard work paid off and things went really well most of the time!

You cannot plan for everything, no matter how hard you try. That's when a large toolbox of interventions comes in handy – it helps you improvise when things go sideways. One night while on this vacation, Jacob felt a storm moving in. These sensitive kids can *feel* barometric pressure changes in the weather like little old arthritic ladies. By morning, he was climbing the condo walls! As soon as I realized it was going to be one of *those* days, I quickly thought ahead, fixed him breakfast on the balcony (where the outdoors could stimulate his visual, auditory and olfactory senses and hopefully fill up that sensory bucket) and gave him a ball of Play-Doh (to engage his tactile sense). We promptly changed plans for that day and enjoyed the indoor pool rather than shopping. Luckily, he was regulating mostly through water that summer, so this was a perfect switch.

You cannot plan for everything, no matter how hard you try. That's when a large toolbox of interventions comes in handy – it helps you improvise when things go sideways.

We *did* eventually go souvenir shopping, however. Stores are full of his triggers (noise, movement and an increase in people), so we prepped him with a visual schedule and went over our "look with the eyes and not the hands" rule (and assigned a parent to follow him at all times). By the time we got to the cashier with our purchases, Jacob still sensed-out. It was too much stimulation all in one place, even for 10 - 15 minutes! He was licking my arm — up, down, up, down, slurp, slurp, slurp — while I waited in line. I got many strange looks, but we kindly redirected his behavior, and while one parent finished the purchases, the other took him out to the quiet car where he could have a snack and drink to help regulate that obvious oral need.

Like Jacob and the shopping trip, my best friend's daughter also had impromptu challenges to overcome. She was even *more* sensitive to routine changes than Jacob, and she especially hated surprises. Well, when you end up at the perfect spot during mini golf to watch the mighty volcano belch smoke and make loud booming noises, let's just say she didn't think it was cool! Her mom reached right into her toolbox and pulled out deep pressure techniques to calm that startled nervous system, and her dad helped a ton by making all of us laugh with a perfectly timed air-guitar solo. Our quick and positive reactions helped right the sensory wrongs, but the best part was seizing the opportunities to teach them introspection and self-regulation ideas for next time. Both sensational kids got better at recognizing their own needs and knowing what to ask for to settle their own nervous systems, and now vacations are not nearly as time-consuming to plan.

Our quick and positive reactions helped right the sensory wrongs, but the best part was seizing the opportunities to teach them introspection and self-regulation ideas for next time.

Holidays provide more opportunities for you to adjust your expectations, plan for success and teach your child to be mindful as well.

Before Jacob's diagnosis, we attempted to divide these special days with both sides of the family, which often meant we tackled three houses in one day (including both grandparents' and ours), and more time spent on the road than with either family. That schedule is exhausting for the most neurotypical of us. After his diagnosis, we chose to adjust our holiday expectations and plan for success. We now see one side of the family on the actual day of celebration and the other side on a day close to the holiday. Each year we switch it up so it is fair to all families. Not everyone likes this plan, but it works much better for Jacob and his needs (it spreads out the transitions, people and excitement so he can stay better regulated at each visit). We also usually pack a sensory backpack full of items for self-regulation, put him in that SPIO suit when he needs it and let him clutch his visual schedule to orient himself on what was coming. Then we pack the softest pjs and heaviest blanket for when he inevitably hits his max.

Thanksgiving time is a specific holiday that taught us how to plan for success. What is hard about Thanksgiving, you wonder? Besides the obvious — a food aversion so strong he has to pull his shirt up and "smell home" every time he passes the kitchen — it is a *fall* holiday. The changing of seasons, plus daylight saving time, can be very difficult for SPD kids (and sensory-sensitive adults). The time change screws up their nervous systems worse than ours. It took Jacob months to get used to seasonal wardrobes, just to have them change again. Dressing and undressing can be a huge challenge for these kids as it involves so much motor planning, requires so many steps, and, for some, throw in sensory sensitivity.

One day Jacob sat on the floor blubbering because he couldn't get his feet in the correct leg holes of long pants. He told me he wished he could just chop his legs off, and he was serious. He had low tone in his hips and core and couldn't sit up straight for a long enough period of time to work one leg (and then the other) into the pants while balancing his body. What did we do to make fall days better? *Plan for success.* We slowly changed his wardrobe over to the next season (he may have worn shorts with a long shirt one day, long pants and a short-sleeved shirt the next) and did lots of hand-over-hand assistance in dressing and undressing to decrease that frustration. Then we worked that body clock back to where it needed to be one day at a time, putting him to bed a little earlier each night. I also carried his lunchbox around like my second purse. It went everywhere, because remember Thanksgiving was smack in the middle of that mess, and this kid didn't eat turkey and dressing.

The scariest holiday to prep for was, of course, Halloween! Navigating the stores with scary decorations that rattle a fragile nervous system was most difficult. Eric and I would shop separately during that season — one parent always kept Jacob at home or in the car for quick trips, while the other took Anna and picked up what we needed. Finding the right costume also required a good bit of cunning. I would buy the softest kind of whatever he requested, and we would spend months desensitizing him to the new piece of clothing. The first day he would hold the costume. The second day he would rub it all over his skin. The third day he would slip legs in and right back out. The fourth day he would put in his legs and arms only for them to come right back out. The fifth day he would wear it for a few minutes. We'd make these day-by-day progressions until he could wear his costume around the house and be comfortable in preparation for Halloween night. When the holiday arrived, we left early to avoid his triggers of noise, movement, and an increase in people, and we followed the visual schedule for the evening's events. Our greatest success strategy of all happened after all of the candy was collected. Jacob would trade the allergy-contaminated candy into the Great Pumpkin (who came every Halloween night) in return for allergy-free candy or a new toy!

Why do we work so hard for success? Because we want our children to enjoy common experiences like everyone else. He deserves to belong, too!

Why do we work so hard for success? Because we want our children to enjoy common experiences like everyone else. He deserves to belong, too!

EXPECT BOOMERANG DAYS

From time to time, my family will be doing what we normally do and planning for success ... clipping along making loads of good progress ... when out of nowhere regression happens. Why do bad days crop up out of the blue? Sensory processing disorder (SPD) is like a boomerang, that's why! Throwing a boomerang is an art, much like learning to handle SPD. You practice and get really good at sailing the boomerang far from you. It may fly so far away you forget it's out there in its arc — but it does come back to you *always*. The question isn't if it will come back, but whether you get knocked in the head or learn to catch. SPD will always be a part of your sensational loved one. Even if you heal SPD and move from *disordered* to just having occasional sensory sensitivities and challenges, it is still part of what has made your child the person that they are.

Sensory processing disorder (SPD) is like a boomerang, that's why! Throwing a boomerang is an art, much like learning to handle SPD.

Every person on earth experiences bad days, sometimes for no apparent reason! People with sensory challenges are no different. Once when Jacob was younger, he wanted to accompany our new kittens to the vet with the rest of us. He had been doing *great* at the time. I still cautiously adjusted my expectations by finding a vet with low wait times and a small waiting room, and then I planned for success, prepping him with a visual schedule and plenty of sensory diet activities prior to leaving the house. Can you guess what happened next? He got overstimulated *anyway*. When worried dogs started coming into the waiting room (sensory kids can be very receptive to the emotional climates around them), Jacob morphed back into Captain Destructo. When I tried to corral him in my lap — praying they would call our names — he started screaming that I was hurting him. I wasn't even being forceful, but to his suddenly heightened sensory system, the lightest touch probably did feel like searing pain. I called my sister — thank the Lord for family. By the time she arrived to take my monkey away (he was literally swinging off the table and screeching these loud war-whoops in the exam room), he had embarrassed me so badly in front of the doctor I apologized and requested a different one for the next visit. Sometimes our best is not good enough, and it is *not* our fault. It is not *their* fault, either. It's the SPD boomerang flying back upside our head when we least expected it.

Sometimes our best is not good enough, and it is *not* our fault. It is not *their* fault, either. It's the SPD boomerang flying back upside our head when we least expected it.

There were times I would see serious regression, without probable cause. He would begin hitting, kicking, pinching, biting, spitting, snatching, screaming (sometimes in anger, but generally joyous whoops of ear-splitting noise – just because), poking, drumming on every surface and running into everyone and everything like a bulldozer. He would have zero control over his body. Many people encouraged me to give him a good spanking, but they were not charged with the responsibility of looking into those little lost, wild eyes — the eyes I remember from pre-therapy days. They were not the ones who looked into the window-like eyes where you could glimpse the person suffering on the inside from a completely disorganized and inflamed nervous system on overload. This child was *not* a discipline issue. If anything, these bad boomerang days reminded me of where we'd been, and where I don't ever want to be again ... and that was a blessing.

Figuring out *why* he struggles doesn't matter nearly as much as finding the reset button. Therapists really came in handy when we had looked everywhere and couldn't find that magic button! I remember a particularly trying week when Jacob had a high engine for *days*. Nothing calmed him. There was no rest to be had for any of us. I called Mrs. Hannah on a Friday night and told her everything he was doing and what we were doing in response. She recommended doing heavy work, then swinging him in a linear motion while soft music was playing. Even if I hadn't been totally exhausted from no sleep, I *never* would have thought of combining those two techniques in that order on my own ... and the beautiful thing was that it worked like a charm. He actually fell asleep that night under his weighted blanket and my heavy heating pad across his chest. Then I slept, too!

Boomerang days can also be progress *in disguise*, like the analogy of the puzzle being dumped out and reorganized to make a more brilliant picture. I recall a special cousin playdate at our house where Jacob absolutely fell apart every 15 minutes. I continually carried him out of the fray and tried to help reset his nervous system. I rocked him. I breathed with him. I explained to him (and the others) what they needed to do so everyone could have fun. We did heavy work and swinging to calm down and reset. No matter how I threw it, that blasted boomerang came right back at us. He was completely spent by the time his cousins were picked up. He needed a good shower and Epsom salt bath, and two hours later, in his favorite pair of two-sizes-too-small zip up footie pjs (nothing gives a little body deep pressure like second skin pjs after all) he *finally* fell asleep.

This was an intense boomerang day, but it showed progress, none-theless. Jacob had *attempted* turn-taking with his favorite swing, *tried* to participate in what his peers were doing, and he was *learning* to cope with thoughts and emotions that his brain previously had no room for. I asked him how he felt when he woke up the next morning. I'll never forget how he rubbed his sleepy eyes and took time to *think* about my question. He finally murmured, "I feel like a firework. A green one. A dark green one, with a little bit of light green." This thoughtful and sensitive boy, who was simply trying his best to fit into this world, was the boy I had been fighting through SPD to see.

He finally murmured, "I feel like a firework. A green one. A dark green one, with a little bit of light green." This thoughtful and sensitive boy, who was simply trying his best to fit into this world, was the boy I had been fighting through SPD to see.

Take time to breathe and steady yourself to throw that boomerang again. Never give up on your sensational kid. Just keep fighting for change one day at a time. Know that these days will be in the mix. You will get tired. You will feel pulled in every direction. There will be days you do not have any patience left, and you lash out in despera-tion. But also know there are silver linings through them all. It's going to be okay in the long run. Just keep throwing the boomerang.

SPECIAL KIDS STILL NEED DISCIPLINE

Kids with sensory processing disorder (SPD) are not responsible for behaviors caused by a hidden handicap, right? Well, the truth is even though they are not responsible in the sense they didn't *mean* to "misbehave," we, of course, still have to correct them so they learn appropriate ways to behave. The root word of discipline is *disciple*. God charged us with the massive job of *teaching* these children the ropes of life. It's great to learn how to meet their needs and plan for success — but when maladaptive behaviors *do* occur, the game plan changes. Discipline first, then meet needs and prep for future success.

It's great to learn how to meet their needs and plan for success — but when maladaptive behaviors *do* occur, the game plan changes. Discipline first, then meet needs and prep for future success.

Discipline in our house takes mostly the form of logical consequences. If you don't do what I've asked, you don't get what you want. Period. You must follow directions in a respectful way in order to get the privileges that follow. If you do not follow the rules or show respect, there will be appropriate consequences to help teach you the importance of thinking first and choosing a different behavior.

For example, when Jacob was about 4 years old, I remember sitting in the doorway of his room refusing to let him out before he threw all his toys into his large bin. He cried that he was hungry. I told him that he needed to pick up his toys first and then we would talk about food. He cried that he needed to potty. I reminded him that he better pick up his toys quickly so that he can make it! It took time and effort to teach him that he *must* follow directions to get *his* freedom, but once the lesson was learned, we had an easier road ahead.

Nowadays, our battles are all about managing screen time with all of its neurological complications. It's really important to *me* that he takes brain breaks and gives his nervous system time to rest and explore the real world. It's really important for *him* to play games and relax from the expectations of the real world. If I have given Jacob a visual list of activities, set his timer, had him repeat them back to me so I know he comprehended, and then he still lost his temper when it's time to get off, he also loses himself the next loop of screen time. Sure, he didn't *mean* to lose his temper, but losing his screen time in addition is a huge motivator to think ahead next time and work harder to control himself. There have been times we've taken weeks of screen time-outs to teach this lesson. With enough practice, he *will* start thinking ahead and choosing less-damaging behaviors, especially as he gets older and matures.

You might hear your SPD child say things like, "But I can't help it!" Jacob pulls this one out often, and the vast majority of the time he is right! He really *can't* help some of the things he does because of how his brain and body work. However, sensory processing differences are neither going to define nor excuse us in life. Once he tried to feed the cats and knocked over the bag of food on accident. I told him it was okay, and he could clean it up. He had a tantrum. He didn't want to … he couldn't … he wasn't going to. Tantrums have the end-goal of changing the parent's mind on something so the child can get their way. However, when he saw I wasn't backing down on the clean-up request, he spiraled into a full sensory meltdown. He was anxious about picking up the cat food because of the smell and texture — scooping it with a cup to feed the cats twice a day could be managed … touching it with his fingers to clean up a mess was repulsive to the point he gagged and nearly threw up. Parents of sensory kids have to be good detectives so they know how to discipline most effectively. Once I understood his source of rebellion, I was able to coach him through pulling his shirt over his nose to "smell home," and I handed him a pair of tweezers. He knew he wasn't going to get to do anything else until he picked up the mess he had accidentally made so there he sat for 20 minutes picking up cat food piece by piece. Sensational children still have to be trained up in the way they should go. We do them no favors in life if we don't teach them that there are consequences to their behaviors and choices.

Sensational children still have to be trained up in the way they should go. We do them no favors in life if we don't teach them that there are consequences to their behaviors and choices.

Jacob is a kid with special needs, but he is a kid *first*. We *all* have challenges. We all make mistakes. We all have to learn to follow rules and be responsible members of society, adults with a moral sense of attitude, behavior and character — or else we suffer consequences we'd rather not bring down upon ourselves. Where the special needs add an extra layer is that we must also afford them the opportunities and tools to manage their *own* lives with their own special challenges. My favorite tool to "help him be good" was in-home reward programs. This is not the same thing as bribing. This reward system requires the parent and child to set goals, and the child works diligently for the desired reward. Don't you set goals as an adult and work hard to attain them? We all do! There were many times I wanted to pull my hair out over one behavior or another — implementing consequences left and right — when all I needed was a reward program. Our mantra was *"Stop and think. Look and see. Is this the best choice for me?"* When he was motivated to work towards a reward, he was more able to stop and think before acting!

That all being said, discipline doesn't work well without a loving relationship and a sense of belonging in the home. When you have instilled those two pivotal pieces, a mutual respect follows. We do a lot of teaching in our home about our value system and how that figures into our attitude, behavior and the actions that make up our overall character. When you talk with your children about such things, you communicate that you think they are smart enough to understand it and worthy enough to rise to the occasion and achieve it. Then, when parents *do* have to discipline, the child knows it is because they are loved, and their parents want the best for them.

EDUCATE THE WAY THEY LEARN

Thankfully, educational choice — whether you choose public school, private schools, cottage schools or homeschool — still lies in the hands of the parents. I hope the rights of parents' choice for critical elements like learning are never taken away. Eric and I *planned* to put our children in public school. All four of our parents worked for the local school system, and we had gone through a public education with great success. There was a time I actually defined Jacob's success with the goal of mainstreaming him into a "regular" school with his sister, but I am eternally grateful that our sensory processing disorder (SPD) journey curved us in a new direction. Through our struggles and inevitable failure in the public classroom, our eyes were opened to other ways of educating children that actually fit our family better all the way around. Our lives are so much richer because we chose to homeschool.

Through our struggles and inevitable failure in the public classroom, our eyes were opened to other ways of educating children that actually fit our family better all the way around.

Annabelle could have made a traditional school setting work, but Jacob was not built for the standard classroom, and the schools and teachers that would have tried to handle him were woefully unequipped. When he was first diagnosed, we sought out a private school that exclusively taught special needs children. We put him in 3-year-old preschool and had monthly team meetings with his teacher and the special needs staff. Our goals were social skills and the ability to follow directions. He did adapt to following routines, yet he couldn't tell me about his day ... not one single thing. His teacher likened him to being in a shell — happy to play by himself or next to another child, but not really *engaging* with them. I was baffled. At home with cousins and friends, he was quite the opposite. Mrs. Hannah and I decided there must be underlying sensory issues inhibiting his growth in a school setting, so we went to work figuring out what was the problem.

A pediatric audiologist found that, in addition to the basic stress of being in a classroom with so much noise, movement and people (and trying to constantly regulate through those triggers), Jacob was hearing all sounds at the *same* level. It was like radio stations blaring different music at the same volume and none of the individual lyrics make it through the noise. No wonder he could follow routines from visually watching the other kids line up for bathrooms or see it was time to eat lunch and clean up, but still not be able to tell me what happened that day. He had no clue, because he couldn't make sense of all the noise. If this wasn't startling enough, I volunteered in the classroom and often noticed him rocking and singing the ABCs to himself when all the other kids were learning colors, shapes and numbers in circle time. This type of "stimming" behavior is most often seen in autistic children. It is a way to self-soothe or stimulate themselves by creating order through predictable and repetitive behaviors, especially when assumed chaos is all around them.

If I had allowed this kid to go to a traditional setting school — public or private — he would have been put into a contained classroom … a classroom for slow learners and behavioral cases. My kid was neither. Parents know their children best, and that's why we chose to homeschool. I knew Jacob would learn best in a familiar, comfortable home classroom of two students with short days, rather than an unfamiliar, unpredictable classroom of 30 kids with long days. The option of schooling around our therapy schedule also afforded us the opportunity to finish up the Interactive Metronome and brain training programs during his preschool and kindergarten years. Taking school slowly, without a set schedule and academic pressure to perform, allowed him to develop at his own pace. By first grade — completely unassisted by occupational therapy or any other intervention program — he suddenly grew in leaps and bounds like he had been catapulted forward!

If I had allowed this kid to go to a traditional setting school — public or private — he would have been put into a contained classroom … a classroom for slow learners and behavioral cases. My kid was neither.

At home, I could tailor our lessons to his needs, making every concept come off the page and into his hands through various activities that incorporated his senses. He learned to recognize his alphabet by giving tangible refrigerator magnets to each of his stuffed animals who asked for a certain letter. He learned letter sounds by pairing them with American Sign Language hand signs. Counting and multiplication tables were taught while jumping on the trampoline and listening to math songs. He learned his spelling words by throwing and catching a ball back and forth in rhythm, saying a letter every time we caught the ball. He naturally became interested in history and science and could rattle off facts that adults have long forgotten or never even knew. He read *all the time,* and still does to this day. He carries books around, loving them to worn and crinkled edges, like adults carry their phones in their back pocket.

Writing was the most difficult subject to tackle because of his fine motor delays, but we worked slowly and at his pace with that one, too. I scribed most of his work from preschool through second grade, but by third grade we saw another burst of ability. He could write just about everything he needed to on his own, and by fourth grade he was unassisted. We also choose to take a standardized test at the end of each year, and it always shows him being ahead academically of typical peers. Homeschooling was addictive for my family, because it was *our* path to academic and personal success. What is yours?

Homeschooling was addictive for my family, because it was *our* path to academic and personal success. What is yours?

There are many ways for a parent to advocate for their child and ensure that they get a quality education. Educating your child the way they learn is an art. First you have to figure out *how* they learn. Annabelle turned out to be a visual-auditory learner, which means she can read and do follow-up worksheets, committing things to memory easily by merely seeing and hearing them. Jacob was full-on kinesthetic — sensory and tactile learning was his goldmine. If your child can function well in a public or private school and that is the best fit for your family, there are a lot of pros to having a team of teachers and administrative staff help plan their education and provide social experiences. There are also special accommodations and individualized education plans you can use to advocate for the needs of your child when you go that route. If school at home is a better fit, there are plenty of pros (and just as many social opportunities) that route as well.

I researched several different homeschooling philosophies, learned about my state laws and what would be required of us, and joined as many homeschooling communities I could find in my physical area and online. I also built a cooperative organization (co-op) from scratch with my best friends which now services both neurotypical and special needs students. When Jacob was in the third grade, we added a cottage school (certified or retired teachers offering a la carte classes to homeschoolers) where they could get a taste of a traditional classroom once a week with a teacher other than me and a classroom of peers. Jacob had a few struggles, again because of the abundance of triggers and academic expectations from another teacher, but the cottage school worked with me and we made it a successful experience with open communication of his needs and sensory-smart strategies like customized visual schedules and sensory fidgets to aid attention and coping skills.

Don't be afraid to branch out and learn your options. Educate yourself first on what *can* be done, and then be courageous to jump in with open eyes and a willing heart. Raising the adults of tomorrow is a high calling. Advocate for your children and see that their needs are met, and most importantly that they can taste success, no matter how you choose to do it.

CALLING ALL EDUCATORS

Whether you teach in a traditional school, cottage school or homeschool, there are many sensory-smart strategies to help your students focus and attend to their lessons (and help you have relaxed, happier days, too)! With permission from the parents and/or administrators, give these tips a try.

If you have a motor mouth or a kid who chews clothing:

- Cut a pack of straws in half and let them chew on a straw.

- Allow them to chew gum (or have parents purchase "chewy" tubes or chewelry necklaces for them to bring to class).

If you have a mover-and-shaker or touchy-feeler:

- Give them a visual schedule of expectations to follow and check off as they finish a task to help keep them focused.

- Provide sensory fidgets to keep those hands busy. Homemade stress balls made with balloons and rice work nicely.

- Encourage them to hug themselves tightly or squeeze their hands together multiple times.

- Replace chairs with exercise balls or let the child stand and do their work.

- Turn their chair around backwards so they straddle it and lean their chest on the back of the seat to do their work at their desk.

- Allow the child to sit in a bean bag chair or lay on a rug to do their work.

- Attach an exercise band to the bottom of their chair so they can bounce and swing their feet without disturbing other students.

- Have them push on a wall to "hold the classroom up" for 20-30 second intervals.

- Have them crawl (hands and knees or bear crawl on hands and feet) to sharpen their pencil and then back to their chair.

- Let them carry heavy books to the front desk. You can send them back later to pick them up when they need another trip!

- Create comic strips dictating behavior choices and how it makes people around them feel when they choose this behavior. This can help a child "stop and think" before acting.

If you have a kid in La La Land:

- Say their name or touch their shoulder and achieve eye contact before speaking.

- Have them repeat directions back to you. If they can't repeat them, they didn't process them.

- Move them close to your chair or desk to cut down on surrounding noise.

- Give them a visual schedule of expectations to follow and check off as they finish a task to help keep them engaged.

- Get them moving with ideas from the section above to "wake up" their nervous systems.

If you have an anxious, sensitive type:

- Write a visual schedule on an index card of what their day looks like and tape it to their desk. It can be generic and laminated for all-year use. Often times, just knowing the plan helps relieve anxiety and calm the nervous system.

- Give them five- to ten-minute warnings before transitions so they can prepare themselves.

- Have a pair of noise cancellation headphones for the hallways, bathrooms and lunchroom.

- Create a quiet space under a desk or in a corner and make up a signal for the child to use when they need to settle themselves and "recharge their batteries."

- Allow them to do work in a quiet, less populated area like the hallway, perhaps with earbuds.

Sensory-smart ideas for the hallway and recess:

- Create a sensory path experience in the hallway(s) that will "fill up" students' sensory buckets through purposeful movement before they sit and attend to academic tasks. (In a traditional school setting this would be most beneficial placed in the main hallway coming into school in the mornings, or the hallway leading to and from the cafeteria.)

- Encourage bear crawling or crab crawling to the next destination.

- Encourage students to safely walk backwards or sideways up and down the stairs while holding the railing.

- Have your students play tug-of-war.

- Encourage swinging, climbing, stomping, and sliding during recess (if on a playground, you can designate an "up" slide to climb up in addition to the "down" slides).

FIND YOUR TRIBE

Have you ever heard the old saying: "It takes a village to raise a child?" Well, I believe it takes the right tribe to maintain your sanity through a journey like sensory processing disorder (SPD). Eric and I had to find the right tribe of doctors, therapists and support networks to keep our family healthy mentally, physically and emotionally ... and good friends who "get it" to keep our world spinning in a positive direction. Because, I learned firsthand, how easy it is to spin out of control without them.

The medical field was a minefield, until I found my tribe. The pediatricians who took care of my children as babies did not know enough about SPD to identify red flags or offer useful advice. I repeatedly shared troubling behaviors of Jacob's with them. I told them how Jacob could not play by himself ... how he couldn't sit still ... how he was rough and wild, *all the time*. I was not exaggerating. We desperately needed help.

During one doctor visit, Jacob got tired of my unending sob story, and he started hitting my legs and crying hysterically. He was only 2 years old at the time. To my surprise, the doctor forcefully took him under the arms, sat him down across the room and scolded him sternly, telling him he wasn't *allowed* to hit Mommy, and he was in time-out. Then she wheeled back around to me with these know-it-all eyes and said, "*That's* how you discipline. Do it consistently and he'll stop a lot of this." You talk about someone being heartbroken and their blood boiling at the same time! I could have reminded her that I was a behavioral therapist before having children and that I knew how to effectively discipline. If she had been listening to anything I had said, she would have realized this troubling trend went deeper than a parenting issue. But instead, I chose to gather my sensed-out child and walk out, conscious to request a different doctor on subsequent visits. That was not the only situation that office mishandled during my time there, however. Her colleagues downplayed the importance of avoiding potential allergy foods and tailoring nutrition when I first wanted to try omitting gluten, dairy and dyes. Then they *continued* to push allergy shots, even when the new diet nipped illness — and seasonal allergies — in the bud once and for all.

I left that toxic environment and found an excellent pediatrician that supported diet and biomedical intervention. He and his colleagues were humble, honest, kind and, most importantly, good listeners. They openly admitted that they did not know everything about SPD, but it was not beneath them to learn alongside me. They welcomed the opportunity to be our medical home base, while we outsourced most of Jacob's healthcare to the integrationist I was already working with closely. The biggest blessing was that the partner of the office gave me his personal email and told me to keep him informed. He was *interested* in the plan, and he cared. I transferred my children's medical records immediately, and they've been wonderful members of "Team Jacob" ever since.

I left that toxic environment and found an excellent pediatrician that supported diet and biomedical intervention. He and his colleagues were humble, honest, kind and, most importantly, good listeners.

I also joined my local SPD support group. I was the only one in my personal circle that had even heard of SPD or sensory processing challenges. It was a lonely experience in the beginning, and I needed people who intimately understood the battle. Being with people who "get it" allowed me to catch my breath from all the explaining I had to do with every other person I encountered in a day ... like the librarian who kept giving my child their famous prune-faced, evil-eye because he was playing hand-drums on every surface, or the grocery cashier waiting impatiently for my 3-year-old to pick up every heavy item and put it on the conveyor belt. At the support group meetings, these people were all at different mile markers on the collective journey. One mother had an older child and knew of interventions I hadn't heard of, while another had a child who just graduated from college proving success *could* be attained. And then there was a father who had a toddler and was scared to death of the unknown, and I had a few experiences to share that would help him get his bearing. A knowledgeable and supportive tribe can teach you so much more than just effective SPD intervention; they can teach you how to walk the journey with courage and contentment.

A knowledgeable and supportive tribe can teach you so much more than just effective SPD intervention; they can teach you how to walk the journey with courage and contentment.

One of the group leaders once said, "You just have to keep it ugly. There is not enough time in our lives to sugarcoat everything. It is really better for everyone if you just have the guts to peel back the layers and show people who you really are, and how it is really going."

Special needs tend to weed out your friend garden. The ones that can handle it tend to stay and bloom alongside of you. The others get uprooted and carried away in the wind, and one day you look up and realize they're not there anymore. This tribe taught me how you can't worry about the opinions you can't change. You have to let go of the anxiety of proving yourself, and your child, worthy of respect and love. When you find people that accept you and your sensational family, you suddenly swell with the courage and peace of mind needed to press on. That's what a support group is for — to support you in the hard times. If you do not have such an organized group physically near you, there are many groups online that can provide you the same feeling of connectedness. You could also start your own group in your community. People fighting the same battles *are* out there; you just have to find them.

People fighting the same battles *are* out there; you just have to find them.

Supportive family and friends, organically rooted and grounded by you from the beginning, are also such a blessing. Our extended families were pretty open-minded and learned about SPD with us. They also worked hard to adjust their own expectations and interactions with Jacob accordingly. Small gestures, like putting allergy-free candy in his Easter basket and Christmas stocking, meant *so much* to us. It allowed him to eat what he was given, like every other kid in the room, without having to switch it out for safe food first.

Good friends are also a must. My two best friends love my children as their own, and I am blessed to have a whole church of loved ones that would do anything for us — day or night. That type of charitable commitment is a gift from above. God *knew* we would need others who understand the different aspects of living with special needs, and be there for the ups and downs of the daily walk. He put them right in my path to find like glittering jewels. Find *your* tribe in every way possible; it will make such an uplifting difference!

LOOK FOR THE GOOD, ALWAYS

Our attitude is what has made us a sensational family, individually and collectively. *Look for the good, always* is our constant philosophy. Philippians 4:8 (King James version Bible) says it best: "Finally, brethren, whatsoever things are true, whatsoever things are honest, whatsoever things are just, whatsoever things are pure, whatsoever things are of good report; if there be any virtue, and if there be any praise, think on these things." Looking for the good smooths the jagged edges that cut us and keeps us framing everything in a positive light.

Like the old philosophy of yin and yang, where light cannot exist without darkness or joy without sadness, a person's strengths cannot exist without their weaknesses.

For every con of Jacob's sensory processing disorder (SPD), there is an equal pro. Like the old philosophy of yin and yang, where light cannot exist without darkness or joy without sadness, a person's strengths cannot exist without their weaknesses. Here are some examples of how we looked for the good in the darkest days of SPD:

- **Visual Sense:** Jacob can be distracted by things most of us don't notice — like dust floating in the sunlight or a shiny letter on a book — but he also can see things we are too busy to look for such as pennies in the grass or a tiny spider building a gorgeous web between two flowers.

- **Auditory Sense:** Jacob is scared when he hears normal sounds that we tune out daily. He cannot function again until we identify the sounds, whether it be the quiet buzzing of a fluorescent light or a lawnmower in the distance. However, his supersonic ears hear the most beautiful things, like wind chimes on a neighbor's porch several houses down.

- **Gustatory/Olfactory Senses:** Jacob has a love-hate relationship with scents and flavors, which makes well balanced dinners and wearing perfumes difficult. But he is an honest critic. Even Anna will watch for his reaction to a new food before she picks up her fork!

- **Vestibular/Proprioceptive Senses:** My boy is a mover and shaker that craves intense interaction. Self-regulating these needs is probably the most difficult challenge we tackle. However, in an event full of wallflowers, he will always be the first to get the party started.

- **Emotional Sense:** Jacob has trouble identifying how his behavior affects other people and how to appropriately communicate his feelings. For instance, when you say you are sorry for hitting Sissy for the 100th time, you have to make your face look sad for her to feel like you mean it. But the little guy also has a deep heart that feels every emotion to its fullest, without the slightest reservation. Jacob smiles as if he never loses and frowns as if he never wins.

Despite the obvious challenges, SPD molded Jacob into a truly sensational kid in so many ways, and because we have adapted to fit his needs, it has made us sensational alongside him! Eric and I work daily to see the world through Jacob's eyes, and not only does it heighten awareness of our surroundings, but it teaches us how to live in the moment. Annabelle would have been a sweet, kind and helpful person regardless, but having a sensational brother enhanced even her views of the world. She was trained as a mini therapist alongside me and being part of the intervention process taught her to be keenly aware of others' struggles. She is the first child on the playground to run to someone's rescue, whether it is someone that got hurt or an underdog targeted by a group of bullies. She is the last to leave a friend in distress until she is absolutely sure they have been comforted. She watches for the person who is having a bad day, and she is always ready to encourage and love them through it. The attitudes of love, acceptance and being each other's soft place to fall are woven into the very fabric of our family life.

The attitudes of love, acceptance and being each other's soft place to fall are woven into the very fabric of our family life.

Every child needs this kind of positive framework to build their lives upon. They need to be loved unconditionally and have their strengths pointed out more than their weaknesses. They need to be told daily that their life has value and that they were created for great purpose. In fact, they don't just *need* this in their lives, they *deserve* it.

One of my favorite reads was Mary Sheedy Kurcinka's *Raising Your Spirited Child: A Guide for Parents Whose Child is More Intense, Sensitive, Perceptive, Persistent, and Energetic.* The spirited children she spoke of mirrored our SPD kid. She admitted that spirited children have unique challenges and take much more energy, patience and flexibility to parent, but she never once referred to them in a negative light. She urges her readers to embrace their differences and help channel them into positive outlets.

It takes a multitude of people with different strengths and sensitivities to make this world go around. For example, my sensory seeker could grow up to be a great construction worker, fireman or trauma doctor. But if he grows up feeling like his very nature is full of negative traits, he will spend his life denying himself in an effort to fit into a box he was never made for. While we have worked diligently to heal the *disorder* that handicapped Jacob's quality of life, we have never wanted to change his *nature*. In fact, we guarded it for we love the person he was made to be.

Allow sensory differences to wrinkle your life and change how you think about things. Let these sensational people teach you how to see the world in a new light. Then in return, teach them to maximize their strengths, minimize their weaknesses and look for the good in *themselves*.

Allow sensory differences to wrinkle your life and change how you think about things.

LOVE EVERYONE THE WAY THEY NEED TO BE LOVED

If *"look for the good"* was our first family motto, then *"love everyone the way they need to be loved"* has become our second. There have been many times that Annabelle has felt deeply jealous of the attention Jacob gets. This was especially true when she was younger and didn't understand as much about sensory processing disorder (SPD) and *why* her little brother required so much attention and effort. There have been many times he has hurt her in one way or another, and she had to be the bigger person —helping us teach him what was right or wrong — which has sometimes felt like an injustice. We have been very open with both of them about SPD and what it means in our family. They know that we *all* have personal challenges of one kind or another, but the important thing to remember is that we were all especially placed in this life together, to help one another. We may not all be treated equally, but we will be treated *fairly* in the sense that everyone gets what they need to succeed.

They know that we *all* have personal challenges of one kind or another, but the important thing to remember is that we were all especially placed in this life together, to help one another.

We raised and loved Annabelle just as fiercely as Jacob, but in a completely different way. When we taught Jacob to recognize and verbalize his own needs, we also taught Anna the art of introspection. He is an extrovert and often needed to regulate his emotion by being with people who supported him. She is an introvert and needed to learn how to sneak away and recharge her batteries by doing favorite activities alone in her room or up a tree in the yard where she was sure to be undisturbed. Where Jacob communicated everything through incessant talking, Annabelle communicated deeper emotions through writing. We started a mother-daughter journal, and when she was particularly overwhelmed with something in life, she'd slip the journal under her bedroom door for me to read and write back in. After several exchanges, she would eventually come back to center and emerge from her safe haven feeling heard, validated and ready to move on. They learned the same important lessons about self-regulation and communication but applied them to their own personalities.

Annabelle also became more responsible at a younger age, so she got the privileges that went along with that level-head and controlled body. When Jacob hit the same age, it didn't automatically mean he would inherit the same privileges. We came to learn that it was okay to treat them differently as long as everyone got what they needed to succeed! They both had strengths to maximize and weaknesses to minimize — which holds true to this day — and they needed to be taught they are distinctly *different*. They needed to grow up knowing who they are and who they can be, and know that both of them are beautiful.

They both had strengths to maximize and weaknesses to minimize — which holds true to this day — and they needed to be taught they are distinctly *different*.

Loving each other the way each needs to be loved also means that we continuously work hard to stay connected as a family unit. In addition to doing activities and outings together, Eric and I also take the kids on individual date nights. Our hope is that they learn that everyone matters, and there is a place for them in this world and in our family. No matter how they need love, we have to give it in a way that they can receive it which looks differently for all four of us. In our family, Eric and Jacob value competence and feeling needed. Annabelle and I value being cherished and having our feelings validated. Eric and I also work diligently on keeping the communication lines open between us, as husband and wife, so we can be the best parent team for our children and the best spouse for each other. When we really get to know one another and respect each need, happiness in the home is very attainable.

LOVE YOURSELF

Creating a sensational home by meeting the needs of your family is very important, but it hinges on you learning to love yourself and meet your own needs in the process. Surely, you've heard the advice flight attendants share prior to departure. If the cabin loses pressure, you must put the oxygen mask on yourself first before helping (or possibly saving) a loved one. I believe that is sound advice for parents of kids with sensory processing disorder (SPD) too. There have been many times when I have felt like the plane is going to crash into the ocean of responsibility, and I am going to get sucked under never to resurface.

I wear so many hats each and every day — I am a wife, stay-at-home mom, in-home therapist, homeschool teacher and co-op director. There's not much time left to just be me. The amount of priorities I am called to handle in a day is daunting, especially the worry that goes into shaping the character traits, compassion, self-esteem and intelligence of another human being (or multiple ones at the same time). I am sure you, too, feel overwhelmed by the many hats you wear. It takes courage, patience and love to get through each and every day and a bucket of self-forgiveness each night I go to sleep to rest assured I am not messing it all up. It is an exhausting balancing act to be the mom who needs to comfort and understand, and the therapist who needs to teach and train ... the ever-accessible teacher of all subjects and at the same time be the director who needs five more minutes to finish working. Something always has to give, whether it is a child who needs extra attention and has to wait until bedtime snuggles, or the house work that doesn't get done. How do I make time to love myself? I compartmentalize my responsibilities and work hard to take the breaks I deserve!

I wear so many hats each and every day — I am a wife, stay-at-home mom, in-home therapist, homeschool teacher and co-op director. There's not much time left to just be me.

I organize best with binders, and I have many binders for all of my many jobs. Remember the binder of observations I took to Mrs. Hannah on day one of therapy? I have a binder for doctors and a binder for running our co-op. Each kid has a binder for school work every year. I also write extensive notes on kitchen memo pads, and leave to-do notes in my various binders for when I pick that job up next. Homeschooling year-round helps organize my stress levels as well since we can move at a slower pace and take time off when needed.

Building expectations into our daily routines is another great way I compartmentalize. On co-op days when I help direct a three-hour class of 25 or more students (and their moms), Annabelle and Jacob know the afternoon and evening are mine to prep the next class or event. They are socially maxed and ready for downtime of their own anyway, but they know screens go off at dinner time and they get time with me again to read books as we prepare for bed.

The organization part comes easy to me. Taking breaks does not. The truth is that I feel guilty when I do something for myself. Our busy culture pushes productivity 24 hours a day, and even when you know that is ridiculous, it is hard to change the tide of what makes you feel successful. I constantly remind myself that if I don't care for myself first, I am depriving the people in my life of the wife, mother and friend that they deserve. That consideration makes building in break times a little easier for me. I don't want to give them the washed up, self-sacrificed version of myself. They deserve the best version of me, and so do I. I'm worthy of the same love I give everyone else.

I don't want to give them the washed up, self-sacrificed version of myself. They deserve the best version of me, and so do I. I'm worthy of the same love I give everyone else.

Loving yourself starts and ends with making time to do what you enjoy; what relaxes and rejuvenates you. Some days the kids scavenge for food and have unlimited screen time while I sit in the sunroom and paint a landscape in acrylics. Other days Eric comes home early for me to go out to dinner with friends. Everyone learns how to live without me at their beck and call when I am locked in my room in one of my writing marathons. It is good for them — in moderation — and most certainly it is good for *me*. Don't lose yourself in life. Take time to live it like everyone else gets to do.

FORGET THE NAYSAYERS

Sensory processing disorder (SPD), formerly known as sensory integration dysfunction, is not nearly as well-known as autism, attention deficit (hyperactivity) disorder (ADD/ADHD) and other neurological disorders, even though research has been compiling since the 1960s. The public at large *still* does not generally recognize it. Whether they are ignorant or willfully unbelieving, there will always be naysayers in this world. These are the people who look in from the outside and judge what they do not know. They stare at sensory meltdowns in the store and assume they are bratty tantrums. They make comments to parents that make them feel incompetent and embarrassed. I mean, doesn't the mental conversation that plays on repeat inside our own heads question our parenting techniques enough? We *know* we shouldn't care about what others think or say as they don't know our child, but the heart still seems to feel the sting even when the rational brain knows we are fighting valiantly for the right.

I mean, doesn't the mental conversation that plays on repeat inside our own heads question our parenting techniques enough?

There was a time I complained to Mrs. Hannah about people who didn't understand Jacob and felt we needed to parent differently. She listened and then patiently asked, "Do you truly believe these interventions — this special way of parenting — is what he needs?" Of course, I did! I had seen the interventions work wonders before my very eyes. The journey had changed him, it had changed me, and it had changed our family for the better. Through the darkness it was building all of us a brighter future. We were seeking out the best methods possible to help Jacob be successful, even though they went against the accepted grain. I had to give myself the permission to let go of the worry about others' opinions and parent in the best interest of *my* family. Even still, I yearned for people to understand us. I guess we will always crave approval and acceptance because we are human. We all appreciate validation over criticism.

I had to give myself the permission to let go of the worry about others' opinions and parent in the best interest of *my* family.

SPD doesn't fit nicely into any box, and you can't always understand it yourself. So how do you help others get it? Or should you even try? I've often wished people could walk one *day* in our shoes. I would pick a really good one, when it was obvious that Jacob's brain and body did in fact process things differently. For example, they could experience the day we went to the funeral visitation for a family friend. I prepped Jacob for the new experience all day long. He had his visual schedule. He had his sensory bucket at the just-right level when we went in, but there were a lot of people and the flower fragrances mixed with food smells were immediately overwhelming for him. People were grieving, and he could feel their pain in his own special way. He began by processing it all well, but after a few minutes his SPD created a traffic jam in his brain and all was lost. He stopped making eye contact, started bumping into our legs while making big arm circles and began making a loud siren sound and turning in circles himself. It happened in *seconds*. By the time we dragged him outside he was a limp noodle. His system was so far jammed that he physically could no longer move correctly, not even to walk.

People don't always believe stories, however. Some would still blame this experience on lack of discipline. So, let's take a look at science, then. SPD is a malfunction of the nervous system. To the naysayers I typically explain how his brain does not process the information received from his senses in the same way ours do. I tell them about how he didn't feel pain or temperature or get dizzy until he underwent extensive therapy that rewired his brain. A few of them may realize that feeling pain and temperature are not behaviors to be judged after all. If they are still listening, I may add information about biomedical treatment and how the gastrointestinal, immune and nervous systems affect each other. Then I add how thankful I am that knowledge has evolved as much as it has in this field — and because we caught it early, Jacob has grown up understanding his body, why he is and always will be different and he wears it like a badge of honor.

In sharing our story, my hope is that some of the naysayers will look at themselves or those they love and realize they *have* seen SPD before, and they just now realize it has a name, and, more importantly, it is a real condition and can be helped. What I really want the crowd at large to hear is that *we need you*. The sensational people in your life need *you*. That grandchild, niece, nephew, neighbor, student or friend's child *needs* you. We can reach goals faster with your support.

What I really want the crowd at large to hear is that we need you. The sensational people in your life need you.

At some point, ignorance does become an active choice. Special needs families cut close family members and friends out of their lives for such a stubborn choice. Their attitudes and actions foil parents' efforts to improve life for their child, and their critical attitude degrades self-esteem and confidence. Some parents may feel that they have enough to battle and will refuse to waste time, energy and resources on an additional battle they cannot win. I sincerely hope the naysayers in your life (and unfortunately you will have some) will not put you in the situation of making such a heartbreaking choice. If you are a naysayer and have miraculously read this far, please respect sensory differences and open your heart to a different way of doing things. If you let them, the sensational people around you will change your life, too, for the better.

Hannah's Professional Opinion

What makes vacations so hard for children with sensory processing disorder (SPD)?

All kids have some difficulty adjusting to new environments, but SPD children have more intense reactions and the effects last for weeks or even months. The majority of these children thrive on routine and schedules, because it helps them feel organized and safe. Different environments with unexpected events heighten their senses and challenge their ability to cope, making outings and vacations that much harder. They lose their perception of where things are, what's going to happen or when another transition is coming, and that can feel very chaotic and frightening to an SPD child.

Any other ideas how to help them adjust quicker and enjoy special family time more?

The key for success is letting go of others' expectations and how outsiders may view your child's negative behaviors, and trusting yourself and the intervention you've learned as the parent. It is also ideal to take advantage of the tools given to you in therapy, and plan for solutions to potential challenges. Remember, the sensory diet can travel. Prepping and exposing your child to upcoming events helps regulation. Trying to keep a form of your home routine will make things more predictable. Incorporating sensory breaks into your trip will also help your child adjust, cope and regulate.

Also, the element of surprise is really for the parents' benefit, not the kids', and it will often backfire if you do not tell them about plans up front. If you don't tell about upcoming, new experiences, they can't process the transition ahead of time, and since they didn't have the chance to prepare their mind and body, they cannot regulate once they are there. Knowing what to expect helps decrease the intense excitement, anxiety or anticipation felt by a sensory kid, so they can modulate themselves and avoid meltdowns. If holidays and vacations are not going well, use it as a learning experience to analyze what is driving undesired behaviors, regroup, and just keep trying until you find what intervention and coping strategies work in multiple settings.

I often refer to Jacob's energy level as an engine running "too high." Can you explain the "How Does Your Engine Run?" program that provided our family with this conversational framework?

We did not follow exact protocol in Jacob's case, but in a nutshell the "How Does Your Engine Run?" program helps create awareness of yourself and how you're feeling by identifying if you are in a state of high arousal, just right or low. If you are too high or low it is hard to think clearly. We have to find "just right" to really be functional. We teach this awareness as it relates to a car engine, through pictures of others and their states of arousal, and when a child can identify others' state of being, they are more likely to self-actualize their own arousal state whether it is too high or low. We can then teach them to adjust it back to "just right" through a variety of regulating strategies.

Regulating strategies are very individualized, so an experienced therapist can help you find what can work for your child.

What do you recommend when parents see regression?

Breathe. Regression and bad days are normal. Everyone has low times; it is part of life. We don't always see constant progress. In general, however, regression doesn't last. If it does, read it as clues that there is something else going on that needs to be addressed in order to start up progress again. We never want kids to feel wrong for having a bad day. It is never wrong to feel emotion. Just communicate that bad days are normal. They sometimes throw us off, but it is temporary. Believe in yourself and breathe.

In some instances, isn't it true that periods of extreme disorganization actually mean the child is growing in the right direction?

Growth can come through conflict, absolutely. Remember that through intense therapy and intervention you are shaking things up and making changes in their bodies. This can be scary and overwhelming for them at times. While it will be worth it in the end, you have to work hard to get there. That includes viewing bad days as part of the bigger picture of overall long-term improvements.

How can support networks increase the success rates for these children and families?

First of all, anyone doubting the need for outside support should check into research on connections in general, and how it is a vital human need. We are social by nature. We need people. More than that, we need connection to people of similar circumstances. It helps us understand we are not alone, which helps us gain strength in so many ways. Secondly, when you connect with people of similar circumstances, they may be able to offer you different intervention tools from their own varied experience. Gaining knowledge and support from those around you is always helpful.

Why is it hard for parents to look for the good when their children are differently abled?

When parents feel the need to control the outcome and have their child be a certain way I think it is based in fear. The parent's perception of what makes a successful person is then projected onto their child; children are an extension of ourselves, so parents may feel they have to put pressure on them to be one way or another. However, you have created an individual, special needs aside, and that child has to grow into who they are, not who you want them to be. If you are afraid of your child being different, figure out what scares you and manage it so they can feel accepted and confident enough to branch out. With special needs especially, it is not about "fixing" them. Even therapists need to look at kids through the lens of educating and developing them into their individual best with the tools given.

Every person has some form of special need. How in your life have you worked to maximize your strengths and minimize your weaknesses?

I have attention deficit disorder (ADD) and have learned how to manage it. My mom created a healthy environment of food and activity (early on I rarely had access to TV or electronics), and I believe that was very beneficial in helping me learn what my body needed so I could function well. I remember one time I was particularly out of sorts and she said, "I don't know what's wrong with you, but maybe you need to go run." Those experiences gave me a mindfulness, a self-awareness and a foundation of skills to help me adapt as I grew into an adult. I remember also thinking I needed to find a job where I would be able to move and wouldn't get bored. I needed something where I could be problem-solving. That's basically what I do all day in OT which is what my body needed. I still have difficulty paying attention at times, but I've learned to recognize it and which strategies work for me to help regain focus. No matter what you do in life, I believe in fostering your strengths and understanding what supports you when you need to minimize your weaknesses.

What is the key to making every member of the family feel loved?

Balance is the key. Your relationships are important to who you are, and you have to keep nurturing them for yourself and the other person(s). Taking care of a child with special needs, who needs more attention, is difficult, and it can feel consuming at times. I urge parents to keep themselves healthy and nurture their family members to do the same. Even if other siblings are not as demanding, learn their cues and be attuned to their needs best you can. You don't want them growing up as their only identity being that of another caregiver in the home, but they need to see that they are also important and worthy of your attention so they can develop their own interests. Teach them to be self-aware, to set their own boundaries within the family dynamic and to communicate their needs when things inevitably get out of balance. It is also important to remember that it can all apply to the health of marriage and being equally sensitive to the needs of your significant other. The overall message is that it is critical to not be so consumed with caretaking that you lose the purpose in your relationships.

How would you choose to educate your child?

I myself am a fan of independence promoted in the Montessori Method of teaching. Life happens fast, and we don't always want to let the kids struggle to learn how to do things themselves (eating, dressing, putting on shoes, cleaning up, etc.), because in the moment when we are rushing to get out the door it is easier to do it for them. We need to let them develop the skills necessary for life, though. We need to slow down and teach them to push past their struggles so they learn what it means to be self-sufficient and successful. Montessori-type schools do this. I am not against public or private school, but if they made changes similar to Montessori, I feel it would really benefit the children.

Formal setting schools seem to have their students sitting at desks most of the day from what I have seen. The benefit is that it can teach attention to sit still and listen, which you need throughout your life, but kids also need to move and interact with their environment. This is another thing Montessori Method incorporates. If formal schools could get kids out in nature and go places where they can learn the academics through experience rather than through memorization of facts in books, they would teach them not only about the world around them but why we want to learn in the first place. As I've mentioned previously, it's always about finding a balance.

Do you have any other words of wisdom on education?

My environment gave me a taste of both worlds, formal school and homeschool. There are pros and cons to both. I advise families to choose wisely and offer a variety of opportunities so that their child is well-rounded. Therapists generally think about the need for social skills, connections, how we learn from others, peers and peer pressure, and tend to lean towards formal school because these things are important. It's one of their first tastes of society. There is a lot of good that comes from formal schooling, so if you homeschool give your children these social experiences too.

I am pretty flexible in my thinking. As a therapist, I see the good aspects of formal school, but I was also homeschooled some through my own education. I understand why some families choose to homeschool. Educational systems today are out of balance in many ways and kids are losing out on learning through experience in so many places. Create a secure environment whatever path you choose, think of what is best for your child and, in the end, find what fits by making sure the goals from both educational worlds are met.

What is your opinion on discipline?

I don't like the term "misbehavior." To me, behavior is a reaction to a given situation, and children are still developing complex communication and learning how to cope, adapt or react appropriately to the world around them. I am always rethinking "discipline" as teaching to the level of what the child can understand at the time in order to help them learn appropriate behavior. As caregivers, it is important to take a breath when behaviors happen that we deem inappropriate — step away emotionally and look at it from where your child is coming from. Try to be objective. That means checking yourself and your own reaction to behavior, so you are not overly emotional in your response. If you can figure out what the child is trying to communicate through their immature or maladaptive behaviors, you are one step closer to teaching them better ways of handling their emotions and reactions.

Now, the exception to that thought process is when danger is present. For example, your child runs into the road. In those instances, an intense reaction (still as objective and neutral as possible, though) on the part of the parent is important. The child needs to know the severity of their actions, and you have to get their attention. If your child has special needs and they cannot cognitively understand the situation and learn from it, then preventative is the best way to go. If they can't stop and think, you have to think and act for them until they are cognitively mature enough to monitor themselves.

Why is it important to address the behaviors first, and meet their sensory needs second?

You do not want to inadvertently reinforce negative behavior with a positive consequence. Let's use the example of if a child gets overwhelmed and reacts with a destructive behavior, like hitting. If you give them deep pressure immediately, they will learn that if they hit, they get their need met. You have to address the behavior first to deter future outbursts, and then figure out what triggers led up to the breaking point (hitting could be their attempt to seek out deep pressure), so next time give deep pressure *before* the destructive behavior occurs. There are always warning signs. It's a matter of learning how to identify them. It is important to teach coping skills and a more appropriate behavior (like asking for deep pressure), then reward them for asking with what will meet the needs. Everything is a learning experience. Parents learn to identify warning signs and triggers, and then they teach their child how to recognize it in themselves. Over time you can teach the child how to listen to their body, use appropriate coping skills and get their needs met so they can grow into functional adults.

How can parents with special needs children better juggle responsibilities and stay sane?

Seek balance in all you do. Balance is so important. Be in tune with your body so you realize when you are getting over-stressed. We want to teach our kids to look for their own triggers, but we have to do the same. We have to understand what sets us off and use appropriate coping strategies before it gets destructive. On the flip side, be careful not to disconnect for too long, and then struggle to reengage. Finding the right coping skills for you is the key to balance.

Also, use your support system so you do not have to do it all by yourself. Delegate and give yourself a break and let those around you feel useful. When you let others help, it shows vulnerability. That is a good example for your child. When they struggle, help them learn that it is okay to reach out and accept help. This is how they will learn to balance themselves as well. Parents are a big influence as children grow and learn.

What would you say to people who do not believe the disorder even exists?

Wait until you have a kid. Seriously. Many parents come in for fine motor issues or another concern and sensory integration problems are not even on their radar. Some people, whether parents or others in their community, do not believe it until they see it personally. SPD presents like mental health disorders in that you cannot see the disorder except through maladaptive behavior. Every SPD case is different, but one thing I know for sure is that I see intervention make changes in behavior.

You can see people passing judgement on families like these. I urge people to understand both sides. Parents do need to teach their kids to respect others and that the world doesn't revolve around them — those are basic life and social skills. But others need to be empathetic. It comes down to respect on both sides. If you are judging another family or child, understand it is not your life, and respect them and their choices. If you can't deal with a behavior, remove yourself from the situation. If you are family or friends and can't easily remove yourself, check your own attitudes and behavior, listen to the parents and what they've learned, and be respectful. If you care enough for a family or child, you will learn with them so you can be helpful, not hurtful. Don't make their lives more difficult. Consider reaching out and building a bridge, and everyone will be better for it.

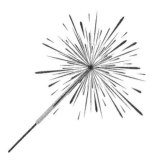

PART FOUR

THE AFTER-STORY AND ACKNOWLEDGMENTS

A PICTURE IS WORTH A THOUSAND WORDS

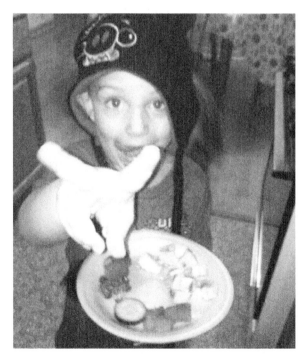

Excited to eat healthy and feel good

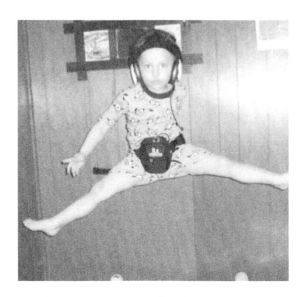

Surviving interactive listening programs

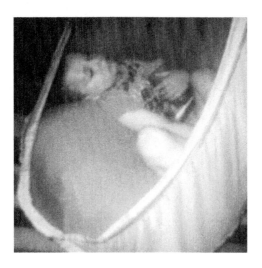

Asleep in his therapy swing

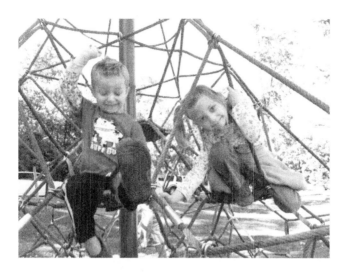

Annabelle, the helpful sissy, with Jacob, the proud bubby

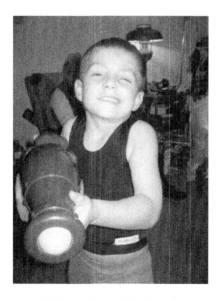

SPIO suit kind of Christmas

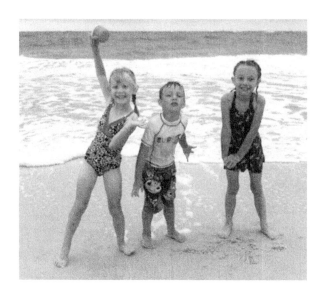

Beach Vacation with Things 1, 2 & 3

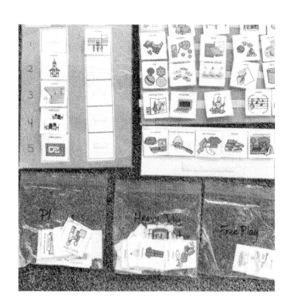

Visual Schedule materials

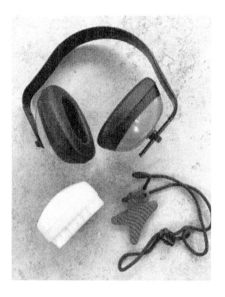

Noise cancelling headphones, chewelry & Wilbarger Protocol brush

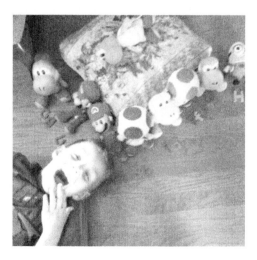

Learning the alphabet with friends

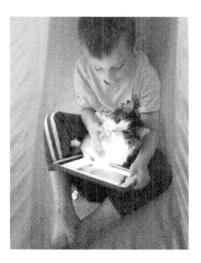

Enjoying a sensory break with his swing and kitty

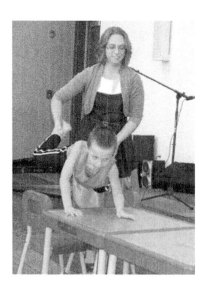

The Strong Man Talent Show Act

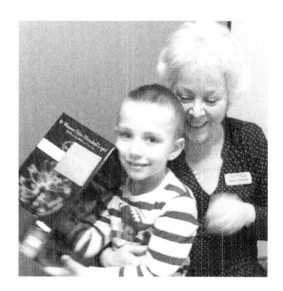

Earning a reward at brain training

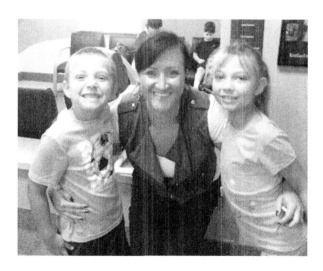

Mrs. Hannah, an answer to our prayer

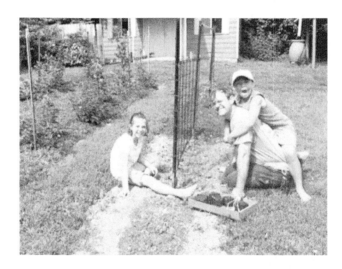

Family heavy work time in the garden

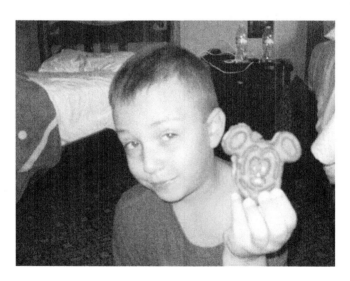

Mickey waffles in Disney World

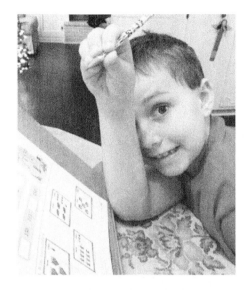

Hooray for the correct tripod grasp while writing

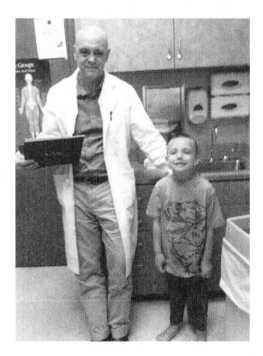

Jacob's amazing Integrationist, Dr. Carl Paige

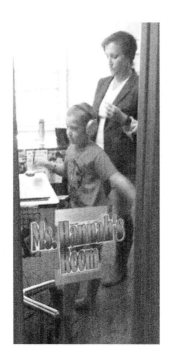

Interactive Metronome session it occupational therapy

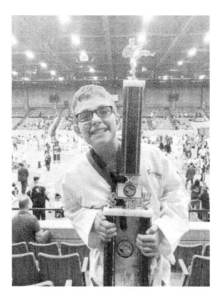

2nd place in forms and breaking

LIFE AFTER SPD

After seven years of diet, biomedical and occupational therapy intervention, Jacob is living his best life and is full of potential. He is still gluten-free, but as his gut healed over the years we've slowly added back in processed dairy (he can handle one cheese stick and yogurt a day, maybe an occasional ice cream — but too much or just straight cow's milk gives him a stomachache). He can even have a piece of candy with a touch of artificial food dyes at a friend's birthday party or holiday celebration without having a behavioral reaction, but again we are very careful not to overload him with potential allergens that would set him up for failure. We see his integrationist once a year to keep tabs on his vitamin, mineral and antioxidant levels as Jacob grows and we then adjust his customized vitamin regimen accordingly. The most startling discovery to date is that if his brain health is not appropriately supported, his body will *eat* the linings of his brain cells to get the fat it's deficient in! (Did your jaw drop open?)

Jacob still has a self-restricted diet and cannot tolerate a variety of foods, although we continue to try new things occasionally and consider it a win for him to look at, smell, feel and taste (maybe eat!) something he hasn't before. Another huge win came when he was 9 years old and he asked for a pair of *jeans*. He wears them occasionally, also now tolerating elastic waistband khaki style pants for church and special occasions, but still and probably always will prefer soft shorts and T-shirts — even in the cold months if he can get away with it. As Jacob grows up, Eric and I try to give him responsibility over his own choices as much as we can and keep an open dialogue about what is acceptable and what is not. We do have basic rules — like arms and legs have to be covered in temperatures below 45 degrees, and you have to eat protein before a sweet treat! We won't always be here to direct our children, so giving them (especially Jacob) the tools necessary to live their best lives is a paramount focus of ours.

So what does a typical "day in the life" look like? Jacob gets up and has one hour of screen time before his morning routine of eat breakfast, take pills, brush teeth and dress. He then chooses to play or read before we do some heavy work or purposeful movement to get his body and mind in sync for school. Once settled, he does cursive, spelling, grammar and language arts, then has a 30-minute to one-hour screen break before finishing math, science and geography/history. Lunch and play time come next, then daily errands, extracurricular activities and two more hours of screen time before his bedtime routine of eat dinner, brush teeth, pajamas, read and bed. We go to martial arts twice a week, homeschool co-op every other week and the cottage school on Fridays. He doesn't take his ADHD medicine on the weekends — *yet* he can now sit through two church services on a Sunday with minimal disruption. For the most part, it is a wonderful life and when it gets rocky for whatever reason, we just go "old-school" and pull out tools from our toolbelt … like the visual schedule (now written on paper instead of using Velcro pictures), heavy work, sensory-rich activities, rolling him up in a blanket like a burrito and pushing on him with a pillow. All I generally have to do is acknowledge that I see him struggling on a given day and say, "What can I do to help you feel more comfortable, Bud?" He knows the answers and I trust his insights.

Today, I consider Jacob healed from sensory processing disorder (SPD). If I took him back to occupational therapy, Mrs. Hannah would wave me out the door and send us back to life. He definitely still has strong sensory preferences, sensitivities and daily challenges, but what we handle now is more reminiscent of the attention deficits and hyperactivity of children with ADHD. It's completely *manageable*. Sure, it takes him longer to master tasks with fine motor skills, like zipping up his coat or tying his shoes, but he can figure it out in time. He has delays in executive functioning skills — it takes a little longer to learn new academic concepts, for instance. But once it clicks, he won't forget! Eric and I also have to have various conversations with him to help him understand why his behavior upsets his sister or friend, why an adult got frustrated with him and how to look for clues in others' body language so he can think first and adjust accordingly. There are many days we still get *so* tired or have a stretch of out-of-routine days and he will end up having a full-blown sensory meltdown by bedtime. It's a rare spiral of emotion when he just can't cope any longer, but it does happen occasionally, especially around seasonal changes or time changes.

Today, I consider Jacob healed from sensory processing disorder (SPD).

So then how can I say he is *healed* from SPD? Well, don't we all get sidetracked in life and forget to run an errand or do a chore? Don't we all struggle occasionally to learn a new skill, or sometimes realize that there are skills that just aren't in our wheelhouse of ability? We definitely all misunderstand people or feel misunderstood ourselves and get overwhelmed by life and occasionally break down mentally and emotionally ourselves! That's *typical* life for all of us. When I say he is healed from SPD, I mean healed from the disorder — the neurological brokenness that plagued his very basic functioning and threatened his productive future. The disorder was the unmanageable part that could only be improved through biomedical treatment, occupational therapy, homeschooling and hard work. Life after SPD is just life with typical Jacob, my intense, sensitive, energetic comedian, and Annabelle, my wise, deep-hearted jewel of a person. Eric and I are some of the lucky ones, and I know that.

Jacob's story had to be told so people knew healing was possible. Living a fully functional and wonderful life *is* possible. We did it. You can, too. Wherever you are on your journey, press on with courage, patience and determination. You may have a child with more severe special needs where sensory processing is only a small portion of your battle. Intervention to help sensory processing will still make a difference in the quality of life for you and your family. Remember, sensory integration is the large base that all ideal central nervous system function is built upon. If you want to improve motor development and cognition, you must work to integrate the senses *first*. Optimal functioning is a worthy goal for everyone, and that can mean something different to every one of us. What is your best life? What's the best life for your loved one? There are also more interventions available that we didn't get to or barely got to experience — interventions like pool therapy, hippotherapy and chiropractic treatments. I'm sure the list will continue to grow as more professionals target sensory processing and integration! Don't ever give up hope on your sensational kids. Research interventions, find help and dig in with all you've got. Change can snowball one day at a time.

Jacob's story had to be told so people knew healing was possible. Living a fully functional and wonderful life *is* possible. We did it. You can, too.

So many people helped us on our journey, too many to count. Please know we have appreciated every single family member, friend, neighbor and stranger that has walked a mile with us or stuck with us for the duration. We couldn't have come this far without you.

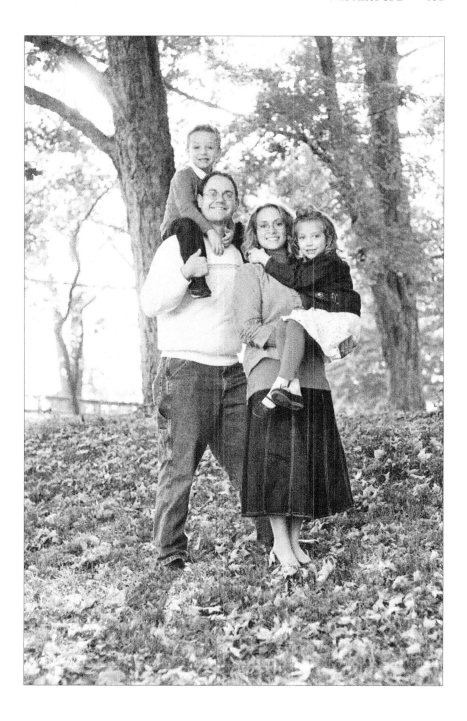

REBECCA'S ACKNOWLEDGMENTS

FAMILY

Throughout the years since Jacob's sensory processing disorder (SPD) diagnosis, I've seen the power of family firsthand. From loving us in our most challenging times to learning about SPD alongside us as we navigated the unknown, I can't stress enough how important it is to have a support system during this journey, and for me, it started with my family.

Eric, you are the best husband and father a family could ask for. God had a great plan when He made us for each other, and there is no one I would rather ride on the roller coaster of life with than you. Thank you for your unending support and encouragement in all areas of my life — from constantly trying new interventions with Jacob to writing this important book — and for sharing your knowledge of all things financial/business-oriented to help make it all possible. Seriously, I am forever grateful for you.

My daughter, **Annabelle**, you are my favorite little girl in the whole wide world — and out of all the little girls in the whole wide world, I would pick you every single time. You are kind, important, sweet and smart, and you have a big heart of gold! You are a Godsend, my love. A brilliant light in people's darker days; the best friend I'll always have by my side. Thank you for letting me write our story down to help other sensational families like ours and for being a huge part of the tapestry of it.

Jacob, you are my favorite little boy in the whole wide world — and out of all the little boys in the whole wide world, I would pick you every single time as well. You are kind, important, sweet and smart, and you make me laugh! You are an amazing person, my love. I'll always be proud of everything you have been, of who you are, and of all you will become. Thank you for letting me write our story down to help other sensational kids like you. Families need to hear our story; other kids will find success because of it. You, my son, are such an inspiration.

My wonderful parents, **Steve and Debbie Duvall**, I'm sure I had my own sensory challenges and quirks growing up and we didn't even know it, but you all loved me unconditionally and naturally helped me maximize my strengths and minimize my weaknesses. You gave me both roots and wings. Thank you for learning new parenting techniques alongside us ... and for the millions of babysitting hours. Believe me, we needed them!

Mike and Carol, you two are the *best* uncle and aunt duo in the world. You all have done more for our family than I could ever thank you for, including encouraging me to publish this book. I'm so proud to be called your niece, and I have appreciated every little gift or act of love, big or small, especially all the yard sale books for my homeschooling library! What a difference each of you have made in our lives.

My sister, **Sarah**, and the cousins, **Ethan, Aubrey** and **Avery**, you all are the graham cracker and chocolate to our marshmallows, the peanut butter to our jelly, and the "chickie" to our "fry-fries." We've raised our kids to be like brothers and sisters, and I've always known you were only a phone call away if I needed you. That's love and commitment on the deepest level.

My in-laws and the cousins, **Rick, Tina, Mark, Jessica, Anthony, Dakota, Tucker and Dominic**, thank you for trying your best to understand why Jacob is the way he is, and why we parent the way we do. I appreciate all the times you tailored gifts to his needs — like soft clothes and allergy-free candy — and for letting the cousins play outside or swim in the pool, the two best places for Jacob to be himself! Your support will always mean more than you know.

FRIENDS

Friends can be found in any and all places, and I feel blessed to have found some amazing ones over the years in communities that saved me in so many ways. From my faith community to my homeschool community — and all others in between — I will be forever grateful for those who lifted me up when I needed it most.

My wonderful **church family**, I can't even begin to single each of you out and tell you what you mean to our family. You know my heart and soul in ways others simply cannot. Thank you for loving our family unconditionally and supporting our journey with Jacob in so many important ways.

My best friends — **Ann Kresen and Ami Koralia** — have proven to me the power of friendship. I am bonded to Ann for life by the understanding and conviction that only comes with special needs children. I've grown together with Ami like two flowers potted by the same gardener. The mental, emotional and physical support as we choose to walk this journey together can never be repaid, and you don't expect it to be. That is the beauty of best friends. I love you both more than you will ever know, but then again, I bet you already do.

There is no place I fit in better than with my **homeschooling tribe!**
The best part, and what I thank you for, is always looking for the good
in my children and cheering them on to reach their fullest potential.
Our lives would have been very different without knowing so many
"Good Friends."

PROFESSIONALS

Navigating a sensory processing disorder (SPD) diagnosis is hard
enough, but when you have a team of professionals that support you
along the way, you feel equipped to tackle each step with confidence.
While we had our fair share of challenges, we landed upon a team of
professionals that were critical to Jacob's success.

Dr. Carl Paige and Dr. Steven Kamber, I firmly believe that getting
the biology in line with how God intended a body to work is the
cornerstone of healing neurological disorders like SPD. Thank you,
from the bottom of my heart, for being experts when I needed them
and friends who understand motherhood. Our journey would not
have unfolded so beautifully if it weren't for you both.

My go-to people in time of exhausting need have been **Hannah
Ragan and the team at Kids Center.** Your expertise was spot on,
and so many positive changes in the right direction wouldn't have
happened without you. Your job is to heal and help us help ourselves,
and when you've done it well — as in our case — we will fade out of
your professional lives and live our own. It's a bittersweet journey,
but know wherever life takes us, you'll always be where our recovery
story began!

The women in **Louisville's SPD Support Group** during the years of
Jacob's diagnosis and intense intervention all offered an emotional
"home base" when I needed one. This group of like-minded individuals took the words right out of my mouth each time I reached out

for help and support. That kind of encouragement is invaluable when you're in the trenches, fighting with everything you have. Thank you for all the honest conversation and knowledge that pointed us in so many right directions.

Last, but certainly not least, **Stephanie Feger and the Silver Tree Publishing team.** You all came in after this story was written, but people wouldn't have heard it without you helping me to tell it. God set our paths in motion toward one another long before we even knew His plans. The unexpected meeting at the mall was no coincidence, Stephanie, as it allowed Him to connect me with the team that could bring our story to the lives of others. Thank you, from the bottom of my heart, for not only making my dream come true, but partnering with me to help others with sensory needs.

Hannah's Acknowledgments

I sincerely thank my husband, family and friends for supporting anything I set my mind to, and to Rebecca for inviting me to work on this important book alongside her. Writing was something I always enjoyed as a child but lost sight of as an adult. If it wasn't for Jacob bulldozing into my life, I don't know when I would have rediscovered it! I'm thankful to be part of such a life-changing experience and to have the opportunity to pay it forward to more families.

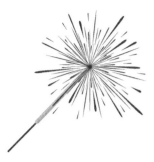

PART FIVE

RESOURCES TO AID YOU ON YOUR JOURNEY

Sensory Processing Disorder Checklist

Quick Ideas for Heavy Work at Home

Books and Websites Everyone
Should Know About

SENSORY PROCESSING DISORDER CHECKLIST

This checklist is not meant to diagnose sensory processing disorder, but rather be an educational tool for your own knowledge in order to help you reach out to professionals who can test for sensory integration dysfunction.

POSSIBLE SENSORY SEEKER TRAITS:

☐ Has an insatiable craving for movement and touch, often in socially inappropriate ways

☐ Is generally loud, needs directions repeated several times, doesn't seem bothered by loud or sudden noises

☐ Wears clothes backward or inside out, doesn't feel light touch

☐ Licks or mouths everything possible, chews fingernails or clothing

☐ Is impulsive to the point of putting themselves or others in danger

POSSIBLE SENSORY AVOIDER TRAITS:

☐ Startles or becomes irritated with unexpected touch, prefers not to be hugged or cuddled

☐ Is generally quiet, distracted by sounds generally not heard by others, covers ears in loud places or with sudden noise

☐ Cuts tags out of clothes and has trouble wearing shoes and/or socks with seams

☐ Is a picky eater and vehemently refuses a variety of foods

☐ Is anxious and cautious to the point of inhibiting social skills and building relationships

OTHER SIGNS OF SENSORY PROCESSING DYSFUNCTION:

☐ Doesn't like playground equipment, or appears clumsy and disorganized while running, jumping, climbing, swinging, playing, etc.

☐ Accidentally spills drinks, knocks things over, slams doors, or uses too little or too much force for the task

☐ Has trouble with simple planning tasks like laying out or folding clothes and getting dressed and undressed

☐ Has trouble with fine motor tasks like writing, zipping or buttoning

☐ Gets easily frustrated or melts down with changes in expectations or during transitions

QUICK IDEAS FOR HEAVY WORK AT HOME

Proprioceptive activities often known as "Heavy Work" are tools to calm, organize and self-regulate the nervous system. You can implement these ideas quickly and safely at home for a quick fix, but remember to reach out to an occupational therapist who can individualize the care and teach you how not to overstimulate the body.

- Push on a wall like you're trying to hold it up

- Walk up and down the stairs forward and backward (alternating feet) and sideways (foot crosses in front and then behind the other each step)

- Play tug of war

- Roll up in a blanket like a burrito and have someone push on you with a pillow from the chest down to your feet

- Lift weights or wear a weighted vest

- Carry a laundry basket or take the garbage out

- Wheelbarrow walk around the room or up and down steps

- Walk or hike with a weighted backpack on

- Bear crawl or crab crawl, add an uneven surface for greater input

- Rough house or wrestle

- Chew on ice, straws or "chewelry" that can be bought for that purpose

- Play with Play-Doh, slime or TheraPutty

BOOKS AND WEBSITES EVERYONE SHOULD KNOW ABOUT

AUTISM/ADD/ADHD/SPD/PERVASIVE DEVELOPMENTAL DISORDERS

- *Unraveling the Mystery of Autism and Pervasive Developmental Disorder: A Mother's Story of Research & Recovery*, Karyn Seroussi

- *Raising a Sensory Smart Child: The Definitive Handbook for Helping Your Child with Sensory Processing Issues*, Lindsey Biel, MA, OTR/L and Nancy Peske

- *The Out-of-Sync Child: Recognizing and Coping with Sensory Processing Disorder*, Carol Stock Kranowitz, MA

- *The Out-of-Sync Child Has Fun: Activities for Kids with Sensory Processing Disorder*, Carol Stock Kranowitz, MA

- *The Out-of-Sync Child Grows Up: Coping with Sensory Processing Disorder in the Adolescent and Young Adult Years,* Carol Stock Kranowitz, MA

- *Thinking in Pictures: My Life with Autism*, Temple Grandin

HEALTHY RELATIONSHIPS/DISCIPLINE

- *Men Are from Mars, Women Are from Venus: A Practical Guide for Improving Communication and Getting What You Want in Your Relationships*, John Gray, PhD

- *Only Love Today: Reminders to Breathe More, Stress Less, and Choose Love*, Rachel Macy Stafford

- *Raising Your Spirited Child: A Guide for Parents Whose Child is More Intense, Sensitive, Perceptive, Persistent, and Energetic*, Mary Sheedy Kurcinka, EdD

- *The New Strong-Willed Child*, Dr. James Dobson

- *Bringing Up Boys*, Dr. James Dobson

- *Have a New Kid by Friday: How to Change Your Child's Attitude, Behavior & Character in 5 Days*, Dr. Kevin Leman

- *How to Talk So Kids Will Listen & Listen So Kids Will Talk*, Adele Faber and Elaine Mazlish

- *1-2-3 Magic: 3-Step Discipline for Calm, Effective, and Happy Parenting*, Thomas W. Phelan, PhD

MEDICAL/NUTRITION

- *Healing the New Childhood Epidemics: Autism, ADHD, Asthma, and Allergies, The Groundbreaking Program for the 4-A Disorders*, Kenneth Bock, MD, and Carmeron Stauth

- *Wheat Belly: Lose the Wheat, Lose the Weight, and Find Your Path Back to Health*, William Davis, MD

- *Grain Brain: The Surprising Truth About Wheat, Carbs, and Sugar – Your Brain's Silent Killers,* David Perlmutter, MD, and Kristin Loberg

- *Glow Kids: How Screen Addiction is Hijacking Our Kids – and How to Break the Trance,* Nicholas Kardaras, PhD

UNDERSTANDING THERAPIES

- *Stopping ADD/ADHD and Learning Disabilities: A Unique and Proven Treatment without Drugs for Eliminating ADD/ADHD and Learning Disabilities in Children and Adults,* Nancy E. O'Dell, PhD, and Patricia A. Cook, PhD

- *This is Your Brain on Music: The Science of a Human Obsession,* Daniel J. Levitin

HOMESCHOOLING/EDUCATION/LEARNING DIFFERENCES

- *102 Top Picks for Homeschool Curriculum: Choosing the Right Curriculum and Approach for Each Child's Learning Style,* Cathy Duffy

- *Right-Brained Children in a Left-Brained World: Unlocking the Potential of Your ADD Child,* Jeffrey Freed, MAT, and Laurie Parsons

- *Teaching from Rest: A Homeschooler's Guide to Unshakable Peace,* Sarah Mackenzie

- *The Unhurried Homeschooler: A Simple, Mercifully Short Book on Homeschooling,* Durenda Wilson

WEBSITES TO GET YOU STARTED

- www.Sensory-Processing-Disorder.com

- www.SPDstar.org

- www.OccupationalTherapyOT.com

- www.SensoryUniversity.com

KEEP IN TOUCH

✉ **Send an email:**

Rebecca@RebeccaDuvallScott.com

HRagan@KidsCenterKY.org

@ **Find, follow and share on social media:**

Facebook.com/Groups/SensationalKidsSensationalFamilies

Facebook.com/RebeccaDuvallScott

Facebook.com/HannahRagan

LinkedIn.com/in/RebeccaDuvallScott

LinkedIn.com/in/HannahRagan

🎁 **Mail or ship something special to:**

Rebecca Duvall Scott
PO Box 934
411 Mt. Holly Rd.
Fairdale, KY 40118-0934

To order books in bulk and learn about quantity discounts:

Send an email! Interested in ordering 15 or more copies of *Sensational Kids, Sensational Families* for your organization, association, conference or to distribute to employees or clients? Inquire at Rebecca@RebeccaDuvallScott.com.

ABOUT THE AUTHORS

REBECCA DUVALL SCOTT

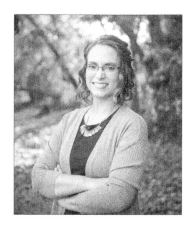

Rebecca Duvall Scott is an accomplished writer, being the recipient of numerous awards throughout her educational career at local, county and state levels. She was awarded the Horrigan's Scholarship at Bellarmine University, where she graduated with a Bachelor's in English. She considered herself a fiction writer, but when her son was diagnosed with sensory processing disorder and she began to blog about her ever-evolving research and his treatment plan, *Sensational Kids, Sensational Families* took root in her heart and this non-fiction memoir was born.

Rebecca lives with her husband, Eric, and their two children, Annabelle and Jacob, in Louisville, Kentucky. In addition to writing, Rebecca enjoys family, church, educating her children at home, painting and directing a local homeschool cooperative organization in which she works hard to accommodate all special needs.

HANNAH RAGAN, MS, OTR/L

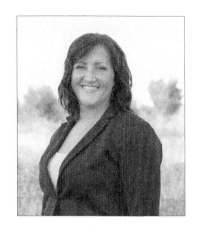

Hannah Ragan, MS, OTR/L graduated from Spalding University with a master's degree in Occupational Therapy. She has worked at Kids Center for Pediatric Therapies in Louisville, Kentucky, for more than 10 years, contributing her expertise within the public school system, outpatient transitional rehabilitation and early intervention home health services. Hannah routinely performs evaluation and treatment of neurological and orthopedic patients with a variety of diagnoses including but not limited to cerebral palsy, spina bifida, brachial plexus injuries, central nervous system dysfunction, sensory and regulatory disorders, attention deficit hyperactivity disorder, learning disorder, pervasive developmental disorder, developmental delay, oppositional defiant disorder, autism spectrum disorders, Norrie disease, Sotos syndrome, Down syndrome, cerebrovascular accident, brain injury and Prader-Willi syndrome. She also has numerous specialty certifications in the area of pediatrics; continues her own education, including intensive training in sensory integration; and has become a fieldwork educator for occupational therapy students from accredited occupational therapy programs.

In her free time, Hannah enjoys running, CrossFit, obstacle races, ballroom dancing, painting and traveling. She is happily married to her husband, Jonny, and together they have one daughter, Zivah, who they adore.

Printed in Great Britain
by Amazon

78341791R00140